Quick Review of
MCI
Screening Test

(Foreign Medical Graduate Examination)

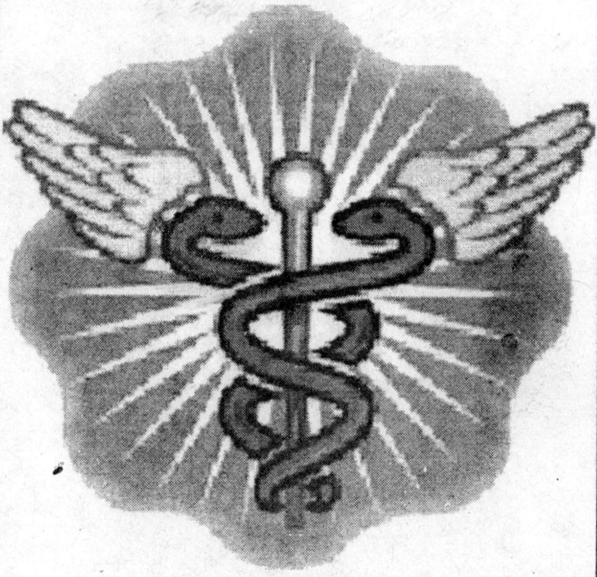

Quick Review of

MCI

Screening Test

(Foreign Medical Graduate Examination)

By

Gouranga Charan Nayak

Sanjeev Kumar

Vijaya Bhanu

Kalaichelvi Gopal

Editor

Chandrasekaran Guhan

PEEPEE

PUBLISHERS AND DISTRIBUTORS (P) LTD.

Quick Review of MCI Screening Test
(Foreign Medical Graduate Examination)

Published by
Pawaninder P. Vij

Peepee Publishers and Distributors (P) Ltd.
Head Office: 160, Shakti Vihar, Pitam Pura
Delhi-110 034 (India)

Corporate Office: 7/31, Ansari Road, Daryaganj
Post Box-7243, New Delhi-110 002 (India)

Ph: 55195868, 9811156083

e-mail: peepee160@yahoo.co.in

e-mail: peepee160@rediffmail.com

www.peepeepub.com

First Edition: **2005**

ISBN: 81-88867-62-4

Printed at
Lordson, C-5/19, Rana Pratap Bagh, Delhi-110 007

truly dedicated
for
MCI Screening Test

CANDIDATES

PREFACE

This book is mainly for the students appearing in the MCI Screening Test for Foreign Medical Graduates. The success in study depends, not only on ability and hard work but also effective methods of study.

This book recapitulates and reinforces the basic techniques of effective self-study and enables the student to get back confidently into the examination groove. A lot many MCQs books are available for students, but they are not available especially for MCI Screening Test.

So our aim is to promote an MCQ book especially meant for MCI Screening Test. In this **Quick Review of Screening Test** we have arranged all the MCQs of March 2005 in subjectwise with explanation. This volume is user-friendly and includes maximum questions of MCI Screening Test March 2005.

We strive to inform you that these questions are based on purely the recall memory of my students who attended the 2005 March examination. The accuracy of some questions may be a suspect but we wish that you have to understand the theme of the question.

Every effort is made to ensure accuracy of material, but publisher, printer, author and editor will not be held responsible for any inadvertent errors.

As you go through the pages of this book, you might come across certain errors and mistakes in the field of grammar, spellings or in the treatment of the subject as a whole. If you find like that critics, please inform us through mail. It will help us to improve our quality.

Please communicate with us:

Gouranga Charan Nayak
guhan_c@hotmail.com

ACKNOWLEDGEMENTS

To our respected guide:

Dr. Vishram Singh
Dr. Satya Narayana

To our teachers:

Dr. Deepak Marwah
Dr. Saswat Roy

To our friends:

Especially

Mr. Rajesh Sharma
(Director of DIAMS)
Mr. Parcha Sundar Rao
(Manager of DIAMS)

To our Colleagues:

Dr. Rahul Singh
Mr. Sargunan Kandasamy

To our Publisher:

Special thanks to:

Mr. Pawaninder P. Vij, for Peepee Publishers and Distributors (P) Ltd., New Delhi

REFERENCES USED

Anatomy	BD Chaurasia Snell; 4th edition
Physiology	Ganong
Biochemistry	Rama Rao
Microbiology	Ananthanarayan
Forensic Medicine	Parik
Pathology	Robbin's
Pharmacology	KD Tripathi; 5th edition
Anaesthesia	Yadav; 2nd edition
Orthopaedics	Maheshwari
Radiology	Review of Radiology by Sumer K Sethi
Psychiatry	Ahuja Batra
Skin (STD)	PM Behlath
ENT	PL Dhingra
Medicine	Harrison; 15th edition Davidson; 19th edition CMDT 2001
Ophthalmology	Khurana
Surgery	Love & Bailey; 24th edition SN Das Manipal Manual of Surgery
Obs. & Gynae.	DC Dutta
Paediatrics	OP Ghai
PSM	Park; 18th edition

CONTENTS

ONE

Anatomy

Q.1. How many arteries and veins present in transeverse section of umbilical cord?

A. Two arteries and one vein
B. One artery and two veins
C. Two arteries two veins
D. None

Ans: (A)

During embryonic period umbilicus have two artery and two vein, but at the age of four month of intra uterine life right umbilical vein disappears and left umbilical vein will be left. Now the umbilical cord contains two arteries & one left umbilical vein & jelly of wharton's. The jelly of wharton is rich in proteoglycan's & function as a protective layer for the blood vessels.

Q.2. The ligament arteriosum is derived from.

A. Ductus venosus
B. Ductus arteriosus
C. Right umbilical vein
D. Left umbilical artery

Ans: (B)

SOME FREQUENTLY ASKED REMANANTS

Ducts arteries	–	Ligamentum arteriosum
Ductus venosus	–	Ligament venosum
Left umbilical vein	–	Ligament teres of liver
Right umbilical vein	–	Disappears
Vitello-intestinal duct	–	Meckels diverticulum's
Wolfian duct	–	Gartner duct

Q.3. No. of segments in liver as per couinauds classification are ?

A. 3 **B.** 4

C. 2 **D.** 8

Ans: (d)

French anatomist couinauds divided the liver in to 8 segments. Each of the segment considered as functional units, each with a separate branch of hepatic artery, portal vein and bile duct & drained by branch of hepatic vein.

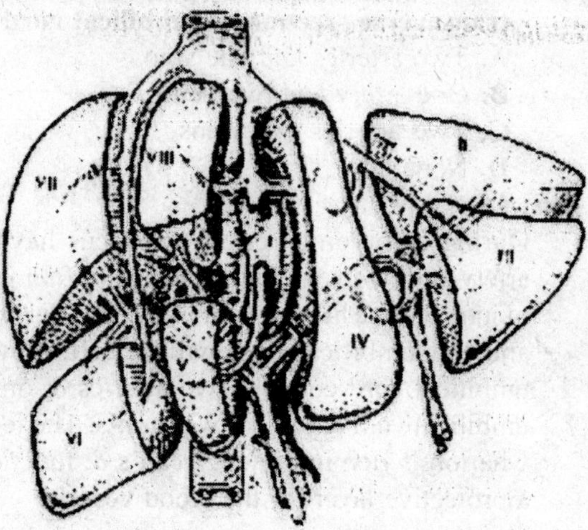

These segments are arranged like in a watch dial from 2'o clock to 8'o clock. The fourth segment is known as quadratus lobe and first segment which situated posterior of the liver which like tail of the liver known as caudatus lobe.

Liver classified as Follows:

Anatomical classification of liver.

Right lobe & left lobe division is by falciform ligament and fissure of ligament teres inferiorly & fissure for ligament venosum posteriorly.

By cantlie's line, liver divided into two equal parts of right and left lobe by line of demarcation through notch edge of gall bladder fossa and to the inferior vena cava posteriorly.

NB: Lungs- each lung have 10 segments. Each segment has its own artery own bronchial. But their veins run in intersegmental plains.

Q.4. The relationship of structures in the costal groove from above and downwards:

A. Nerve, artery, vein

B. Artery, vein, nerve

C. Vein, artery, nerve

D. None of the above

Ans: (C)

Some commonly asked relationship.

intercostal groove – (from above downwards)

- Intercostal **v**ein
- Intercostal **a**rtery
- Intercostal **n**erve

Mnemonics [VAN]

femoral triangle (medial to lateral)

- Femoral **v**ein.
- Femoral **a**rtery
- Femoral **n**erve

Mnemonics [VAN]

Hilum of kidney (anterior to posterior)

- Renal **v**ein
- Renal **a**rtery
- Renal **p**elvis

Mnemonics [VAP]

Cubital fossa (medial to lateral)

- Median **n**erve
- Brachial **a**rtery
- Biceps tendon
- Radial **n**erve

Mnemonics [MBBR]

Popliteal fossa

* <u>upper part</u> (medial to lateral)

- Popliteal **a**rtery
- Popliteal **v**ein
- Tibial **n**erve

Mnemonics [AVN]

*<u>middle part</u> (from superficial to deep)

- Tibial **n**erve
- Popliteal **v**ein
- Popliteal **a**rtery

ANATOMY

Mnemonics [NVA]

*lower part (from medial to lateral)

- Tibial **n**erve
- Popliteal **v**ein
- Popliteal **a**rtery

Mnemonics [NAV]

Q.5. All are the branches of internal iliac artery *except*:

A. Ovarian Artery.

B. Superior Vesical Artery.

C. Medial Rectal Artery.

D. Inferior Rectal Artery.

Ans: (A)

- The ovarian and testicular arteries are the lateral branches of abdominal aorta (at the level of L2 vertebra).
- At the level of L4 vertebra abdominal aorta divides into Right & Left common iliac artery, which subsequently divides into external & internal iliac artery.
- Internal iliac artery divides into anterior & posterior.

Anterior Branches -U^2 V^2PROG

U- **U**mbilical Artery **U-** Uterine artery

V- **V**aginal artery **V-** vesical artery (inferior)

P- **P**udendal artery (internal)

R- **R**ectal Artery (middle)

O- **O**bturator Artery

G- **G**luteal inferior artery.

Posterior branches - I L G (I love god) "Mnemonics"

I- **I**leal lumbar artery

L- **L**ateral Sacral Artery

G- **G**luteal artery (Superior)

NB:

- Left testicular vein drains to left renal vein.
- Right testicular vein drains to inferior vena cava.
- Left supra renal vein drains to left renal vein.
- Right supra renal vein drains to inferior vena cava.

ANATOMY

- Lymph drainage of testis & ovary to para aortic lymph node.
- Lymph drainage of posterior part of cervix to pre sacral lymph node.

Q.6. Muscle which helps to open Eustachian tube while opening the mouth.

A. Palato Pharynges
B. Tensor palate
C. Tensor tympani
D. All of the above

Ans: (B)

- There are 2 muscle which helps to open Eustachian tube. They are tensor palate & levator palate.
- **Try to remember**

Action of muscle of Soft palate.

Levator palate: elevate the soft palate, closes pharyngeal isthmus, open the auditory tube.

Tensor palate: tenses the soft palate & opens the auditory tube.

Palato glossus: pulls the root of tongue & closes oropharyngeal isthmus.

Palato Pharynges: pull up the wall of pharynx & shorten it during swallowing.

Musculus uvula: pulls up the uvula.

NB: All the muscle of the soft palate are supplied by the cranial part of spinal accessory nerve except TENSOR PALATI, which is supplied by the mandibular nerve.

(Reference: SN 6th Edition Page No. 742, BDC 3rd Volume, Page No.-180)

Q.7. The bipolar neurons seen in:

A. Cochlear ganglion.
B. Sympathetic ganglion.
C. Parasympathetic ganglion.
D. Dorsal root ganglion.

Ans: (A)

According morphological classification the neurons are divided into......

- Uni-polar e.g. Dorsal root ganglion.

ANATOMY

- Bipolar e.g. Vestibular ganglion, Cochlear ganglion, Retinal ganglion (VCR).
- Multi-polar e.g. Motor neurons of spinal cord, motor neurons of brain, cilliary ganglion, autonomic ganglion, pyramidal cells and purkinje cells.

NB: *Pseudo unipolar neurons found in*

- Ganiculate ganglion
- Mesenchepalic neuron
- Trigeminal ganglion

***Mnemonics*: Good Morning Teacher.**

Q.8. The inversion and eversion of foot joint at:

A. Ankle-Joint

B. Calcaneo-cuboidal joint

C. Sub-talar joint

D. Inferior tibo fibular joint

Ans: (C)

1. Sub talar joint known as talo-calcanean joint, which is a plane synovial type of joint, it permits for eversion & inversion of foot. It is also done by talo calcaneonavicular joint & partly at transverse tarsal joint is known as talocrural joint.
2. Ankle joint-synovial variety of hinge joint, strengthened by medial (deltoid) ligament & lateral Ligament. Movements are dorsi flexion & plantar flexion.

   NB: the ankle joint is most frequently sprained joint in the body.
3. Calcaneocuboidal joint – it is saddle type of joint.
4. Inferior tibofibular joint is syndesmosis joint.

   (Reference: Clinical Anatomy by Vishram Singh Page No. 156, BDC 3rd Volume Page: 136)

Q.9. Most important Ligament preventing uterine prolapsed:

A. Cardinal ligament

B. Round ligament of uterus

ANATOMY

C. Broad ligament
D. None of the above

Ans: (A)

Classification of Uterine Support

- Primary support
  a. Muscular or active
    1. Pelvic diaphragm
    2. Perineal body (it acts as a anchor of pelvic diaphragm)
    3. Urogenital diaphragm
  b. Fibro muscular or mechanical
    1. Uterine axis
    2. Pubocervical ligament
    3. transverse cervical ligament / cardinal ligament /Mackaenrodts Ligament
    4. Uterosacral Ligament (also one of the chief support)
    5. Round ligament of uterus
- Secondary support: are found by peritoneal ligaments.
  a. broad ligament (has no supportive function)
  b. uterovesical fold of peritoneum
  c. rectovaginal fold of peritoneum

(Reference: 5th Edition Obes & Gyne by J. Willocks & K. Phillips (Churchill Livingstone)

TWO

Physiology

Q.1. Major amount of salivary secretion by:

- **A.** Submandibular gland
- **B.** Parotid gland
- **C.** Sublingual gland
- **D.** Minor salivary gland

Ans: (A)

About 1500 ml of saliva is secreted per day
The pH of saliva 7-8

Gland

Parotid	- 20% of total
Submandibular	- 70% of total
Sublingual	- 5% of total

Saliva contain 2 digestive enzymes, lingual lipase & alpha-amylase

Q.2. All or none law is obeyed by:

- **A.** Spike potential
- **B.** End plate potential
- **C.** Generator potential
- **D.** Action potential

Ans: (D)

Difference between Local Potential and Action Potential

Local Potential	*Action Potential*
Does not follow all or none law	Follow all or none law
Not self propagating	Self propagating
Travels with decrement	Travels without decrement
Can be depolarizing / Hyper polarizing	Always depolarizing

So all other in the options are local potential except action potential. Examples of local potential are EPSP/IPSP, End plate potential, receptor potential, synaptic potential, Generator potential, Electronic Potential

Q.3. Growth hormone is inhibited by:

A. Bromocriptine
B. Exercise
C. Going to sleep
D. Glucose

Ans: (D)

The stimulators that increase growth hormone secretion fall into 3 general category.

1. Conditions such as hypoglycemia and fasting in which there is an actual or threatened decrease in the substrate for energy production in the cells.
2. Conditions in which there are increased amounts of certain Amino Acids in the plasma.
3. Stressful Stimuli

Stimuli that increase secretion.

Hypoglycemia
2-deoxyglucose
Exercise
Fasting glucose
Stressful stimuli
Pyrogen
Various physiological stress
Estrogen & androgen
Going to sleep
L-dopa & μ adrenergic agonist that penetrate the brain

Stimuli that decrease secretion

REM sleep
Glucose
Cortisol
FFA
Growth hormone

Medroxy progesterone.
The response to glucagon has been used as test of Growth Hormone response.
(Ref. 21st Ed of Ganong.Page No. 408)

Q.4. Characteristic for smooth muscle cells:
A. Absence of myosin
B. Presence of sarcoplasmic reticulum
C. Latch state
D. Fixed tension relationship

Ans: (C)

Smooth muscle have no troponin or tropomyosin, but they have actin and myosin.
They have no sarcoplasmic reticulum, No T-tubule.
No Z lines. The contraction is stimulated by extracellular ca+.
Latching - is the characteristic of smooth muscle Even after the dephosphorylation of myosin, the cross bridges continue to attach in the same position for some time. There is no fixed tension relationship.

Q.5. Prolactin is stimulated by:
A. TRH
B. ACTH
C. GNRH
D. Dopamine

Ans: (A)

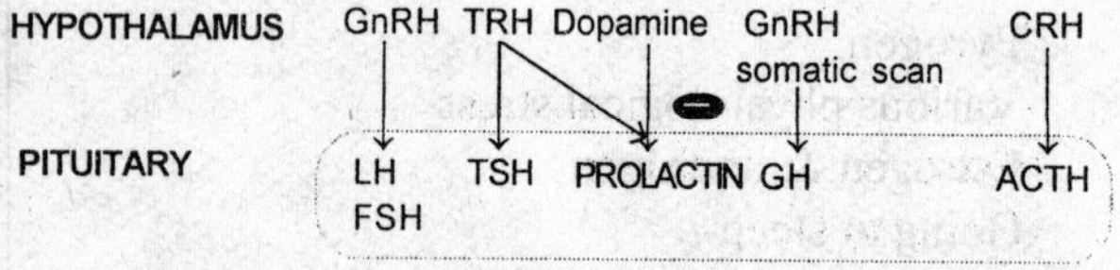

Hypothalamic control of anterior pituitary hormones are mediated by specific hypothalamic releasing hormones. Eg. Thyroid releasing hormone. Exception to this is prolactin secretion which is under inhibitory control of Dopamine. So dopamine inhibit release of prolactin. But TRH, VIP & other polypeptide found in hypothalamus which stimulate prolactin secretion. If transpituitary section done none of the anterior

PHYSIOLOGY

pituitary hormones will be secreted except prolactin because the inhibitory control of dopamine will not be there. Due to transpituitary section releasing hormones will not be secreted into the pituitary.

Other important points:

Oxytocin cause Milk ejection

Prolactin cause Milk secretion.

(Reference: Davidson 21st Edition P.No:687)

Q.6. Brunner's gland is in:

A. Lungs

B. Stomach

C. Duodenum

D. Ileum

Ans: (C)

Brunner's gland is a mucin secreting cells in duodenum. The other mucin secreting cells of GIT - Goblet cells, Crypts of lieberkuhn.

Cell type	*Secrete*
1. Parietal cells (oxyntic cells)	H+ (Hcl), Intrinsic factor blood group substances.
2. Chief cell/peptic cell/ Zymogen cells	Pepsinogen
3. Neck cells	Mucin & HCO_3
4. G-cells	Gastrin

In stomach there are 4 type of cells.

Some glands to remember:

- Bartholin glands-in vestibule.
- Brunner's gland-in duodenum.
- Cooper's gland-bulbourethral gland.
- Master gland-Hypophysis.
- Meibomian gland-modified sebaceous gland present in tarsal part of eye.
- Montgomery's gland-modified sebaceous gland present in areola of breast.
- Rosenmuller gland-Node of cloquet which receive lymph from glans penis in male & clitoris in female.

- Skene's gland-urethral gland which opens to the vestibule on either side of external urethral meatus.

NB: NO GLAND IS PRESENT IN VAGINA.

Q.7. Which has the longest life span?

A. Lymphocytes
B. Neutrophils
C. Monocytes
D. Platelets

Ans: (A)

The RBC	- 120 days.
Lymphocytes	- 100-200 days.
Neutrophils	- 3-5 days.
Eosinophils & Basophills	- 4-8 days.
Platelets	- 8-10 days.

Q.8.. Anterior pituitary secretes

A. ADH
B. Oxytocin
C. FSH
D. GnRH

Ans: (C)

Pituitary gland divided into anterior and posterior

From *Anterior lobe* TSH
ACTH
FSH
LH
GH
Prolactin
B-Lipotropin

From *Intermediate lobe*
Melanocyte stimulating hormone
Lipotropin

From *Posterior Lobe*
vasopressin
oxytocin.

Q.9. Faecal mass mainly derived from:

A. Undigested food
B. Indigested Food
C. Intestinal flora
D. Intestinal secretions

PHYSIOLOGY

Ans: (B)

First we will see - what is the normal content of feces - 70% water, 30% solid.

In solid

1. Cellulose and indigestible fibre - variable, bulk laxatives work by providing a larger volume of indigestible material to the colon - so these make major part of solid.
2. Bacteria 30 percentage of total solid.
3. Inorganic material 15 % of total solid.
4. Fat and fat derivative 5 % of total solid.

Q.10. Normal pH of blood is:

A. 7.26 - 7.36
B. 7.45 - 7.50
C. 7.36 - 7.44
D. 8.32 - 8.56

Ans: (C)

This question is asked many times, so we tried to give you some list of pH.

Urine: 4.5-5.5 (it also varies)
Plasma:7.36-7.4
Pancreatic juice: 8.0-8.5
Saliva: 7.0-8.0
Vaginal secretion: 4.5
Stomach: 1.5-3 (According to food varies)
Tear & CSF: 7-7.2.

Q.11. All sensations carried through lateral spinothalamic tract *except*:

A. Pain
B. Cold
C. Hot
D. Vibration

Ans: (D)

Dorsal column transmits

a. Touch (Fine)
b. Pressure
c. Vibration
d. Proprioception

Lateral spinothalamic tract
a. Pain
b. Temperature
Anterior spinothalamic tract
a. Crude touch
b. Pressures.

Q.12. Which is not interfered at loop of Henle?

A. Na^+
B. Kl^+
C. Cl^-
D. Uric acid

Ans: (D)

In the loop of henle many substances are filtered. Reabsorbed, secreted and excreted, so they interfere in Na+, K+, Cl- , urea, total solute and water.

The loop of henle is not handling the uric acid.

Q.13. The most active form of thyroid hormone at tissue level:

A. T4
B. T3
C. RT3
D. DIT

Ans. (B)

Thyroid hormones enter cells, T3 bind to thyroid receptors in the nuclei. T4 can also bind, but not so avidly, RT3 is inert.

T3 acts more rapidly and 3 to 5 times more potent than T4

Thyroid secrets 80 mg/day of T4
4 mg/day of T3
2 mg/day of RT3

Thyroid binding proteins does not change in hypo & hyperthyroidism.

Thyroid binding protein is increased in the condition like → oestrogen & tranquillisers.

Thyroid binding protein is decreased in the condition like → glucorticoids and androgen.

(Reference: Page No.326 Ganong)

Q.14. Glomerular filtration rate is:

A. 50 ml/min
B. 50 ml/sec
C. 125 ml/min
D. 1125 ml/sec

Ans: (C)

- *GFR in a normal man is 125 ml/min.*
- *Renal plasma flow (RPF) is 700 ml/min.*
- *Effective renal plasma flow (ERPF) is 625 ml/min.*
- *Renal blood flow - 1.2 - 1.3 L/min (420ml/100mg/min).*
- *Liver blood flow - 1500ml/min (58ml/100mg/min).*
- *GFR is measured by inulin.*
- *Renal plasma flow is measured by paramino hippuric acid (PAH).*

(Reference: Page No: 709, Ganong - 21st Edition)

Q.15. Normal glomerular capillary pressure is:

A. 15 mmHg
B. 25 mmHg
C. 35 mmHg
D. 45 mmHg

Ans: (D)

Pressure in renal valves:

- Mean systemic arterial pressure→ *100mmHg.*
- Glomerular capillary pressure →*45mmHg.*
- Glomerulus→*44-42mmHg.*
- Peritubular capillaries→*8mmHg.*
- Renal vein→*4mmHg.*

Glomerular capillary pressure - That is about 40% of systolic arterial pressure.

(Reference: Page No: 707, Ganong 21st Edition).

Q.16. O_2 consumption of heart can be known by:

A. CO
B. HR
C. Fick's principle
D. Sarling law

Ans: (B)

- *The O_2 consumption by the heart is determined primarily by the Intra myocardial tension. The contractile state of myocardium and the heart rate.*
- *Ventricular work per beat correlates with O_2 consumption.*
- *The fick's principle is used to calculate the cardiac output.*
- *Cardiac output can also be measured by the Indicator dilution method.*

Starling law of heart: The length of the muscle fibers is proportionate to the end diastolic volume. The relationship between ventricular stroke volume and end diastolic volume is called the **Frank starling curve.**

(Reference: Page No: 577, Ganong 21st Edition)

THREE

Biochemistry

Q.1. Wheat is Lacking in:

A. Methionine
B. Lysine
C. Both
D. Thiamine

Ans: (B)

Next to Rice, Wheat is 2nd important *cereal* in which deficient amino acids are lysine & threonine, but in Pulses (Legumes) protein deficient in *Methionine*. These amino acids are known as limiting amino acids.

Pulses are also known as poor man's Eat.

Flatulance related with pulses due to rich in oligosaccharide. The ICMR (Indian council medical research recommended 100 gm protein / 1kg body weight.

Soya bean is richest in protein (40%) among pulses

Thiamine (B1)

Important sources of B1–cereals, wheat, gram, yeast.

The 2 principal thiamine deficiency disease are been Beri beri & Wernicke's encephalopathy.

Q.2. Chitin is a polymer of:

A. N-acetyl Neuraminic acid
B. N- acetylated glucosamine
C. N – acetyl galactosamine
D. Aglycon

Ans. (B)

- *N-acetyl Gluosamine* Linked by β (1-4) linkage.

Glucosamine is chief organic of cell wall of fungi. Also constitute of shells crustaceae [crabs, lovsters, etc.], where pt. Occurs as "Chitin" which is made up repeating units N-acetylated Glucosamine so it is a Homopolysacchride. Hence Glucosamine called as Chitosamine.

- N-acetyl Neuraminic acid (NANA) is component of Homopolysacchride cells wall. It is also known as sialic acid. Neuraminidase Hydrolyses split NANA from the compound.
- Galactosamine occurs as N-acetyl galactosamine in a group sulphated mucopolysaccharide. As chondroitin sulphate which present in cartilage, bones, tendons atleast valves. So galactosamine is called as chondrosamine.
- Aglycon—nothing Non carbohydrate residue of Glycosides.

BIOCHEMISTRY

Q.3. Daily required dose of Fe in an adult man is:

A. 0.5 mg
B. 1 mg
C. 2 mg
D. 3 mg

Ans. (B)

According to the age group, the requirement of iron/**day as given below:**

Children (1-12 yrs)	– **1.0 mg**
Adult Male	– **0.9 mg**
Adult female	– **2.8 mg**
Pregnancy (First half)	– **0.8 mg**
Second half	– **3.5 mg**
Lactation	– **2.4 mg**

Most common cause of Nutritional Anemia – **Iron deficiency Anemia**. Iron is mainly absorbed in duodenum & upper small Intestine. M/c organic disorder in clinical Medicine – **Iron deficiency Anemia**.

Cut –off points for the diagnosis Anemia.
Adult Males -**13 gm/dl**
Adult females (Non-pregnant) – **12 gm/dl**
Adult females pregnant – **11 gm/dl**
Most common cause of iron deficient Anemia in adolescent Male →**GI –bleeding**.
Most common cause of iron def. Anemia in reproductive age of female→**Menstrual bleeding**
Hook worm.
India → *Nectar Americans – 0.05ml blood/day/worm*
World Wide →*Ancylostoma Duodonale – 0.2ml/worm/day*
(Reference: Park 18th Edition, Page No. 450)

Q.4. Watson's DNA Models:

A. Left parallel
B. Right Handed Antiparellel
C. Right parellel
D. Linear

Ans (B)

DNA – The large polynucleotide of DNA is organized in the form of *double Helix, (Watson & click).*

Two polynucleotide chains coil around each other in such a way 3-phosphate end of one chain is approximated to the 5' – OH end of the other and the 5' – OH end of the one is approximated to the 3' – phosphate end of the other. If one of the chain is running in the 3'-5' direction, the other running in the 5' – 3' direction – so they are *antiparellel*. Both are *Right handled helices* each coiled around the axis.

DNA of all the cells in the adult human body. If screeched and arranged end to end will have a length of 10^{10} miles. This more than the distance from the earth to sun ($9x10^7$ miles).

(Reference: Page No. 81 Text book of Biochemistry (A.V.S.S. Rama Rao))

BIOCHEMISTRY

Q.5. Niemann-pick disease due to deficiency of:

A. hexoaminadases
B. Glucosidase
C. Sphingomyelinase
D. Galactosidase

Ans: (C)

These are several storage disease like lysosomal storage disease & glycogen storage disease etc. Here we will deal about lysosomal storage disease. This is due to accumulation of specific macromolecules within cells due to deficiency of one or other lysosomal enzymes.

Disease	*Deficient enzyme*	*Stored material*
Gaucher disease	Acid β glucosidase	Glucosyl-CERAMIDE
Niemann – pick disease	Spingomyelinase	Sphingomyelin
Tay-sach's disease	β- Hexo-saminadase A	GM2 Gangliosides
Sandhoff disease	β –Hexosa-minodase A+B	GM2 Gangliosides
Hunter disease	α - L –iduronidase	Dermatan sulphate, Heparan sulphate
Hurler's disease	Iduronate sulfates	Dermatan sulphate
Fabry disease	α – Galactosidase A	Globotriaosyl Ceramide

BIOCHEMISTRY

Q.6. RNA is detected by:

A. Western blotting
B. Southern blotting
C. Northern blotting
D. Crystallography

Ans: (C)

- DNA by southern blotting
- RNA by Northern blotting
- Western blotting is used for HIV virus Antigen [Protein]

Mnemonics:

It may sound's funny – but Easiest way to remember.

<u>S</u>outh people eat <u>**D**</u>OSA
<u>N</u>orth people eat <u>**R**</u>OTI

Q.7. Water Soluble form of vit K:

A. Phylloquinone
B. Fornaquinone
C. Menadione
D. Mephyton

Ans: (C)

You all know friends the vit A,D,E,K all are fat soluble.

There are 3 type of vit K

K1 – phylloquinone – from leaves intestinal
K2 – Fornaquinone – from Intestinal Bacteria
K3 – Menadione – synthetic

The vit K3 is 3 times more potent than Natural varieties. It is water soluble, so it can given parenterally. Vit K1 another name *mephyton or phytonadione*.

So soon after birth, all infants receive a single Intramuscular dose of vit K preparation for prophylaxis. Role of vitamin C: production & regulation of clothing factors.

Vitamin C Stored: IN LIVER.

Q.8. BMR depends mainly on:

A. Surface area
B. Race
C. Sex
D. Climate

Ans: (A)

B M R depends on

1. Surface area
2. Age
3. Sex
4. Climate
5. Race
6. Store of Nutrition
7. Drugs.

But BMR is directly proportionate the body surface. So BMR mainly depends on surface area. BMR is measure in an apparatus called BENEDICT –ROTH Metabolism apparatus.

BMR – A person is under basal conditions if he

is in the post absorptive state (i.e. 12 to 24 hrs after the last meal) physically & mentally at rest in a reclining position. The Metabolic rate under those conditions is called basal Metabolic rate BMR.

For every rise of temperature by 1C° BMR increase 7%

BMR is elevated in HYPERTHYROIDISM.

BMR is decreased in HYPOTHYROIDISM.

Q.9. Ammonia in the brain is detoxified into:

A. Urea
B. Glutamine
C. Glutamate
D. Protamine

Ans: (B)

(Reference: Lippincott's 2nd Edition Page No. 240)

Glutamine–this amide of glutamic acid provides a nontoxic storage & transport form of ammonia. The formation of glutamine occurs primarily in the muscles & liver but also important in the nerve system where it is the Major mechanism for the removal of Ammonia in the brain. Circulating glutamine is removed by kidneys and deaminated by glutaminase

Q.10. T4 is derived from:

A. Histidine
B. Phenylalanine
C. Tryptophan
D. Glycine

Ans: (B)

Phenylalanine gives thyrosine and from thyrosine products are T3, T4, Melanin, Catecholamine (i.e. Dopamine, Epinephrine, Norepinephrine)

Tryptophan gives to serotonin.

Q.11. Final Product of Purine metabolism is:

A. Uric Acid
B. NH3 + CO_2
C. Urea
D. Fumarate

Ans: (A)

The end product of purine metabolism in primates Including man and the Dalmatian dog is Uric Acid. In the lower animals bird and reptiles this is broke down by enzyme uricase to form allantoin.

Some imp. Points

Purine base are = Adenine & Guanine

Pyrimidine bases are = cytosine & Thymine

(Reference: Rama Rao 9th Edition Page No. 327)

Q.12. Unconjugated bilirubin is increased in all *except*:

A. Dubin Johnson

B. Gilbert

C. Criggler-Najjer

D. None

Ans: (A)

Remember

Mnemonics *"GUN"*

G – *Gilbert*

U – ***Unconjugated bilirubin (-)***

N – *Criggler-Najjer*

DR – *Dubin Johnson & Reiter both are increased in Conjugated bilirubin.*

Q.13. Familial hypercholesteraemia is due to:

A. HDL receptor deficiency

B. IDL Receptor deficiency

C. VLDL Receptor deficiency

D. LDL Receptor deficiency

Ans: (D)

Remember:

- Of the total cholesterol absorbed 80-90% is etherified with long chain fatty acids in intestinal mucosa itself.
- When chylomicrons reach with lipoprotein lipase to form chylomicron remnants, only 5% of cholesterol ester is lost and the rest is taken up by the liver when the remnants react with the Apo-E or LDL receptor and hydrolysed to free cholesterol.

- Chylomicrons carry dietary cholesterol to the liver.
- VLDL formed in the liver and transported cholesterol into the plasma.
- VLDL converted to IDL in blood by LPL with removal of TGs from it.
- Most of the IDL changes into LDL by losing their Apo-E and some TGs.
- HDL is synthesized in the liver cells and removes cholesterol from the extra hepatic fissure and transfers it to the liver.

Note:

- Maximum exogenous TGs is seen in Chylomicrons.
- Maximum endogenous TGs are seen in VLDL.
- Maximum TGs is seen in Chylomicrons.
- Maximum cholesterol is seen in LDL
- Cholesterol is transported from liver mainly as VLDL.
- Carrier of cholesterol in plasma is LDL.
- Dietary cholesterol is transported to the extra hepatic fissure by LDL.
- Cholesterol is transported from the extra hepatic fissure to the liver by HDL.

Answer to question:

Hyper lipoproteinemias are 5 types, depending on which type of lipoprotein abnormality.

Table-17.3, page no: 314, Rama Rao.

Type-II, otherwise called as Familial hypercholesterolaemia.

Type-II is most common type.

Type-IV is also fairly common.

Type- I, III, V is rare.

FOUR

Forensic Medicine

Q.1. Haemodialysis is not effective in:

A. Lithium
B. Barbiturate
C. Theophylline
D. Digitalis

Ans: (D)

Haemodialyses is not useful in poison of:
Kerosine Oil
Digitalis.
Benzodiazipines.

Haemodialysis is useful in:
MNEMONICS— **BLAST**
B - Barbiturate
L - Lithium
A - Alcohol
S - Salicylate
T - Theophylline

Q.2. Pin point pupils are seen in all *except:*

A. Organophosphorus
B. Opium
C. Pontine Haemorrhages
D. Dhatura

Ans: (D)

Remember:
Mitotic pupils are seen in
- Carboxylic Acid
- Organophosphorous
- Opium
- Pontine haemorrhages.

Q.3. Lesion with intact skin but internal pathology will be:

A. Contusion

B. Abrasions

C. Lacerations

D. Hypostasis

Ans: (A)

Contusion is an effusion of blood into the tissues due to the rupture of blood vessels (Vein, Arterioles) caused by blunt trauma. In contusion there is a painful swelling and crushing or tearing of the subcutaneous tissues usually without destruction of the skin.

Q.4. Subpoena is a kind of:

A. Decomposed body tissue tribunal

B. Designation

C. Document

D. Court tribunal

Ans: (C)

Subpoena or summons:

It is written document issued by the court and served on the witness under a penalty in all cases by the police officer to attend the court fort giving evidence on a particular day & time.

Q.5. Most informative test in paternity:

A. Finger Printing

B. DNA Finger Printing

C. Blood Group

D. HLA

Ans: (B)

(Reference: Parik 21st Ed. Page No. 386)

Other Application of DNA Finger Printing

- Murder
- Sexual Crime
- Paternity Dispute
- Identification of Mutilated remains
- Extortion Cases
- Identification of bodies in exhumation case.

Q.6. Post Mortem stiffening is called:

A. Rigor Mortis
B. Cadaveric Spasm
C. Livor Mortis
C. Algor Mortis

Ans: (A)

- *Rigor Mortis:* This is a stage of stiffening of muscles with shortening of the fibers.
- *Livor Mortis (Post Mortem staining):* is a bluish purple or purplish red discoloration which appears under the skin of the dependent part of the body after death due to capillovenous distention.
- *Algor Mortis:* Cooling of the body. The curve of cooling is *sigmoid* in pattern.

Cadaveric spasm: In this condition the muscles that are contracted during life become stiff and rigid immediately after death without *the stage of primary relaxation.*

Cadaveric spasm occurs in cases of:

Sudden Asphyxial death.
- Firearm injury
- Drowning
- Excitement fear.

Cadaveric spasm mainly occurs in **voluntary muscles.**

Q.7. Female can give constant for sex if above:

A. 16 years.
B. 12 years.
C. 19 years.
D. 21 years.

Ans: (A)

A man commits rape if has sexual intercourse with a woman with or without her constant when she is **under 16 years** of age.

Exception

- Sexual intercourse by a man with his own wife is not rape, if she is **above 15 year age.**

- A woman of 16 years & abo' e can give valid consent for sexual intercourse.
- Rape offence is punishable under **sec-376 IPC**
- Rape is a cognizable offence.

Cognizable offence: It is an offence in which a police officer can arrest a person without warrant from the magistrate. eg. **Rape, Murder, Dowry Death, Ragging Death due to rash or negligent act etc.**

FIVE

Microbiology

Q.1. Q-Fever is caused by:

A. R. Prowazekii
B. R. tsutsugamushi
C. C. Burnetti
D. Rochalimaea quintana

Ans: (C)

Q-Fever is a Highly Infectious Zoonotic Disease with worldwide distribution. It occurs mainly in person associated with sheep, goats, Cattle or other domestic animals.

Agent: The causative agent is Coxiella Burnetti

Animal Hosts: Cattle Sheep Goats Ticks & Some Wild animals are natural reservoirs.

Mode of Transmission: Q-Fever differs from other rickettsial infection in that there is no Arthropod involved in its transmission to man. The Organism transmitted through Aerosols Inhalation of Infected dust from soil contaminated by urine or feces of diseased animals. The organism can also gain entry into the body through abrasions conjunctivae or ingestion of contaminated food such as meat milk & milk products.

Q.2. Lyme disease is caused by:

A. T. Palladium
B. Burgdorferi
C. B. Recurrents
D. L. Interrogans

Ans: (B)

Lyme Disease:

I.P 3-30 days.

Borreila Burgdorferi transmitted by the bite of Ixodid-ticks.

B. Burgdorferi is a fastidious bacterium, which can be grown in a modified Kelley's (BSK) medium.

What are fastidious Bacteria?

Bacteria which grows in enriched media are called fastidious bacteria's other fastidious bacteria's are:

1. Streptococcus Pneumoniae
2. Streptococcus Aureus
3. H. Influenza

Q.3. VR (Venkataraman Ramakrishnan) Media used for:

A. V. Cholera
B. *E. Coli*
C. *Streptococcus*
D. Shigella

Ans: (A)

Venkatraman Ramakrishnan (VR) medium is a transport medium for Vibrio Cholera (Stool Specimen).

Cary blair medium is also a transport medium for vibrio cholera.

Cary Blair Medium is a universal transport medium. It is also suitable transport medium for salmonella & shigella.

Other Important transport Medium.

Transport for **streptococci – Pikes Medium**

Transport Media for respiratory specimens-**Stuart Medium**.

Q.4. All are dimorphic fungi *except*:

A. Cryptococcus Neoformans
B. Blasto Mycosis
C. Coccidioidomycoses
D. Histoplasmosis

Ans: (A)

C. Neoformans is a yeast-unicellular capsulated fungus.

C. Neoformans is most common cause of meningitides in AIDS patient.

Cryptococcus Neoformans is readily demonstrates in CSF by:

- Direct Microscopy
- Culture O_2
- Serological tests for capsular antigen

Direct Microscopy

Unstained wet preparations of CSF mixed with a drop of India ink demonstrate the capsule of C.Neoformans.

Stain such as Alcian blue & Muccicaramine stain the capsular material.

Culture: Cryptococcus can be easily culture from the CSF on Sabarouds Agar.

Remember: It has four serotypes A.B.C. & D. Most infections are caused by A&D.

Some important points about other fungal diseases:

Pityriasis Versicolour is caused by Malassezia furfur (Pityrosporum orbiculare)

Diabetic patient have an increased incidence of candida infection:

The commonest culture media used in mycology is sabouraud's glucose Agar.

- Trichophyton causes infection of Hair Skin & Nail.
- Microsporum Caused Infection of Hair & Skin.
- Epidermophyton causes infection of skin & Nail.

Q.5. Bedside rapid urease breath test is diagnostic of:

A. *H. Pylori*

B. Proteus

C. Klebsiella

D. Staph Aureus

Ans: (A)

H. Pylori is a gram-ve spiral flagellate bacillus. It is a noninvasive lives in mucus overline gastric mucosa (Its strange, that is lives in gastric mucosa but causes duodenal ulcer).

H. Pylori is *Micro-aerophilic*

H. Pylori infection
↓
Superficial gastritis
↓
Hyperacidity → Duodenal Ulcer
B. Cell lymphoma
Chronic Atrophic Gastritis → Non-Cardia Gastric Adenocarcinoma

Diagnosis

Various test used are:

- Serological test – Detection of antibodies against H. Pylori
- Urea Breath test
- Biopsy based tests:
  - Biopsy Urease test
  - Histology
  - Culture

Serological test for H. Pylori are the simplest test involving assessment of specific IgG level in serum. Its major drawback is that. It cannot be used to assess the outcome of T/T as serum antibody titre take at least 6 months to decrease

C^{13} or C^{14} Ureas breath test:

- It is a rapid noninvasive test.
- Unlike serological test, Urea breath test can be used to asses the outcome of T/T 1 month after its completion.

Recommended 7 to 14 days regimens for the eradication of H. Pylori.

Ureas +ve organisms.

- Proteus.
- Klebsiella.

- Staph aureus.
- Cryptococcus
- H. Pylori.
- H. influenza.
- Diptheroids
- Ureaplasma Urealyticum

All Myco bacteria (Typical and Atypical) except MAI (Mycobacterium Avium Intracellulare)

Q.6. Which is Gram + ve?

A. Fusobacterium
B. Bacteroids
C. Bartonella
D. Erysipelothrix Rhusiopathiae

Ans: (D)

Some Important Points:

Bartonella are Gram –ve. Bacilli usually transmitted by arthopods. Which Invade endothelial cells & Blood cells

Human Pathogenic strain is B.Bacilliformis, B. Quintana & H. Henselae.

Cat Scratch Disease is caused by Bartonells henselae.

Bacillary Angiomatosis- IN which vascular Nodules or tumours appears on the skin. Mucosa & other locations. This disease is seen more commonly in HIV infected & other immunodeficient persons.

The genu fusobacterium contain long thin or spindle shaped bacilli with pointed ends. F. Nucleatum is normal inhabitant of the mouth & is found in oral infection.

Bacteroides are gram-ve anaerobic bacilli.

Bacteroides are the most common anaerobes isolated from clinical specimen

Some important point

All bacilli are gram – ve except **MALDAC** (**M**ycobacterium tuberculosis, **A**nthrax, **L**isteria, **D**iptheria, **A**ctino myces, **C**lostridium tetani)

All cocci are gram + ve except Neisseria Morexella.

E. Rhusiopathiae is a slender, nonmotile, nonsporing, non capsulated, gram + ve rod. It causes swine erysipelas and *Human Erysipeloid.* Human infection usually occurs on the hand or fingers of persons handling animal, fish or animal product.

Q.7. Paragonimus Westermani is commonly called as:

A. Lung fluke
B. Liver fluke
C. Intestinal fluke
D. Blood fluke

Ans: (A)

Parasites which migrate to Lung / Sputum examination is useful in

MNEMONICS:

SHAPE **S** = Strongyloides
H = Hook worm
A = Ascaris
P = Pargonimus, westermani
E = Echinococcus
(if secondary infection of lung occur)

Parasites which do not migrate to lung/absent in sputum:

WPW
W = Whipworm
(C Trichuris Trichuria)
P = Pinworm (Enterobius)
W = Wucheria Bancrofti

Important Point

- Fasciolopsis Buski is the largest intestinal fluke.

Classification of trematodes on the basis of their habitat.

Blood trematodes

In vesical venous Plexus⇒S. Haematobium

In Rectal Venous Plexus & Portal venous plexus ⇒S. Man Soni & S. Japonicum

Hepatic Trematodes ⇒F. Hepatica, C. Sinuses

Lung Trematodes ⇒P. Wester Mani

Intestinal Trematodes

Small Intestine⇒F. Buski, H.Heterophyes, M.Yokogawi, W. Watsoni
Large Intestine⇒G. Hominis.

Q.8. Promastigote form of Leishmania seen in:
A. NNN Medium
B. Spleen
C. Bone
D. Lymphnodes

Ans: (A)

Leishmania Donovani

It is an obligate Intracellular parasite of reticuloendothelial cells predominantly of liver, spleen, bone marrow & other vertebrate hosts (dogs and hamster)

Morphology

The parasite exists in two Morphological forms
- Amastigote
- Promastigote

Amastigote

In the amastigote form the parasite resides in the cells of reticuloendothelial system (Macrophages, Monocytes, Polymorphonuclear leucocytes or endothelial cells) of vertebrate hosts.

Promastigote

Are found in the digestive tract of Insect vector & in the culture media.
Culture media for Leishmania are
- NNN Medium
- Hockmeyers Medium

Promashgote form is the infective form
Indian Kala-azar is considered to be a non-zoonotic infection with man as the sole reservoir. Important sandfly hosts include. P. argentipes, P. Orientals & P. Martini of these P. argentipes is the Indian vector.

Q.9. Staph. Aureus is a normal inhabitant of:

A. Nose

B. Throat

C. Skin

D. All of the above.

Ans: (A)

10 to 30% of healthy people carry staphylococci in the nose

10 % of healthy people carry staphylococci in the Perineum and Hairs.

Other important point

The human Nasopharynx is the only reservoir of the Meningococcus.

Q.10. Babesiosis in India most commonly transmitted by:

A. Hardticks

B. Softicks

C. Mites

D. Sandflea

Ans: (A)

Hard ticks transmit the following diseases

- Tick Typhus (Rocky Mountain spotted Fever)
- Viral Encephalitis (eg. Russian spring summer)
- Viral Fever (eg. Colo rado tick Fever)
- Viral Hemorrhagic Fever (eg KFD in India)
- Tularaemia
- Tick Paralysis
- Human Babesia

Soft tick transmit

- Q- fever
- Relapsing fever
- KFD

Remember the table by heart definitely you will find questions from this **table page-574, Park 18th edition.** Arthropod-borne disease.

(Reference: Park 18th Edition Page No. 586)

Q.11. The sabin Feldman dye test used to diagnosis:

A. Toxoplasmosis
B. Crytosporiodium
C. Rubella
D. Isospora Beli

Ans: (A)

The sabin Feldman dye test depends upon the appearance in 2-3 weeks of antibodies that will render the membrane of laboratory cultivating living T. Gondii impermeable to Alkaline methylene blue. So that organism are unstained in the presence of positive serum.

Imp. Point about T. Gondii

- Infection is transmitted through encysted organism by eating infected raw or uncooked meat or through contact with infected cat faces. It can also be acquired across placenta.
- The most common congenital defects are deafness, cardiac malformations and cataracts.
- Other resulting defects include glaucoma, retinopathy, microcephalus cerebral palsy, IUGR, hepatosplenomegaly, mental & motor retardation.
- Congenital Infection is considered to have occurred if the infant has IgM rubella antibodies shortly after the birth or if IgG antibodies persist for more than 6 months.

The gestational age at which maternal infection occurs:

The first trimester is most disastrous time for fetus. As the organs are developing infection in the second trimester may cause deafness. But those infected after week 16 suffer no major abnormalities.

Age of gestation	*Overall risk of damage to fetus*
< 11 weeks	90%
11-16 weeks	20%
17-36 weeks	0 %

Acute infection is diagnosed by detecting IgM specific antibody. High level of IgG antibody titre & detection of seroconversion from IgG from negative to positive.

Treatment:

Pyrimethamine 25 mg orally daily + oral sulpha diazine 1 gm four time a day is effective.

Pyrimethamine is not given in the first trimester.

Spiramycin 3 gm orally daily has also been used as an alternative.

Q.12. Toxic shock syndrome MC caused by:

A. Staphylococci
B. Streptococci
C. S. Pneumococcus
D. None of the above

Ans: (A)

(Reference: Anathanarayan Page No. 196/ 17th Edition)

Toxic shock syndrome toxin is potentially a fatal multi system diseases presenting with fever hypo tension, Myalgia, Vomiting, Diarrhoea, Mucosal Hyperaemia & an erythematous rash, which desquamated subsequently.

TSST-I – Most strains belong to phage group I

- It is formerly known as *enterotoxin* for *Pyrogenic exotoxin* is most often responsible.

Staphylococcal enterotoxin & TSST-I are super antigens which are potent activators of T Lymphocytes.

Remember

Streptococcal toxic shock syndrome is caused due to release pyrogenic exotoxin or erythrogenic exotoxin.

These toxins are produced only by a few strains of beta haemolytic group A streptococci.

Dick test

It is a test used to identify children susceptible to scarlet fever.

MICROBIOLOGY

Q.13. Crescent shaped gametocytes seen in:

A. P. Vivax
B. P. falciparum
C. P. Malariae
D. P. Ovali

Ans: (B)

Schyffner's dot in RBC – **P. Vivax**
Maurree's dot in RBC – **P. Falciparum**
Ziemann's dot in RBC – **P. Malariae (Rosette shaped merozoite)**
Jamese dot in RBC – **P. Ovali.**
Ring & crescent shaped gametocytes are seen in **P. falcifarum**
M/c type of Malaria in India seen - **P. Vivax.**

Q.14. A child after consuming a food in a party complaints of vomiting & diarrhoea after 6 hrs. the diagnosis is:

A. Staphylococcus Aureus
B. Bacillus cereus
C. V. cholerae
D. Salmonella.

Ans: (B)

1-6 hrs.
- Stap Aureus
- Bacillus cereus

8-16 hrs.
- Cl. Perfringes
- B. Cereus

>16 hrs.
- V. cholera
- EHEC
- ETEC
- Salmonella
- Shigella
- Cl. Botulinum.

(Reference: Park (Page No. 178 & 179) 16th Edition)

Q.15. Organ which undergoes involution:

A. Heart

B. Adrenal Gland

C. Pancreas

D. Thymus

Ans: (D)

- **Involution:** The return of a enlarged organ to its normal size.
- **Incase of thymus:** It is the first organ in animal species to become predominately lymphoid.
- In human being the thymus reaches its maximal relative size just *before birth.*
- It continues to grow fill about the 12th year.
- After puberty it undergoes spontaneous progressive involution; it functions best in early life.
- It located behind the upper part of the sternum.
- Thymus has two lobes. In Digeroge syndrome there is thymic aplasia.
- Like thymus, pregnant, uterus also goes under involution (after delivery).

(Reference: Anantnarayan, Page No. 117-118)

SIX

Pathology

Q.1. Amoebic ulcer is:

A. U-shaped
B. Undetermined edges
C. Flask shaped
D. Everted edger

Ans: (C)

For Explanation refer the Question No.31 in surgery (perforation of typhoid usually occurs during 3rd week).

Q.2. Longitudinal ulcers are seen in:

A. Tuberculosis
B. Typhoid
C. Amoebiasis
D. Malaria

Ans: (B)

For explanation see the surgery Question No.31 (perforation of typhoid usually occurs during 3rd week).

Q.3. Minimal Change GN all are true *except*:

A. Loss of foot process
B. Normal Basement membrane
C. Lipoid Nephrosis
D. Poor response to steroids

Ans: (D)

Minimal change dose (MCD) also known as - Lipoid Nephrosis which is most common cause of Nephrotic syndrome in children.

Main feature is **loss of foot process**, under ***electron microscope***

It gives good response to **steroids**.

Note: Loss of Foot process can be seen under electron Microscope .Under light Microscope those will be no change. M/c cause of nephritic syndrome →IgA Nephropathy **(World wide).** It is known as **Berger's disease.** ***Spike & dome pattern in subepithetial*→Membranous GN.**

Q.4. Ovarian tumours most commonly arise from:

A. Sex cord
B. Germ cell
C. epithelial cells
D. stroma

Ans: (C)

Most common ovarian tumor→epithelial cell (60%) Tumor

Most common ovarian tumor with pseudo-myxoma peritonei→mucinous cystadenoma.

Most common epithelial cell tumor →serous cyst adenocarcinoma. (In serous cystadenocarcinoma psammoma bodies are seen)

In Granulosa cell Tumor →call exner bodies

Endodermal sinus Tumor → schiller duval bodies

Hilus cell Tumors →Reinke's Crystal.

Q.5. HIV affects:

A. CD 8
B. CD 4
C. Macrophages
D. B+C

Ans: (D)

HIV infects CD4 mainly and also macrophages, dendritic cells.

In India most common Strain of HIV-I (subtype c)

Most common malignancy in AIDS patients **Kaposi sarcoma**

Most common fungal infections in AIDS patients **Cryptococcus Neoformans.**

Most common blindness in AIDS patients **CMV retinitis**

Most common space occupying lesion in AIDS- Toxoplasmosis.
(Reference: Page No. 231 Robinson. 7th Edition)

Q.6. Which of the following is not Premalignant condition:

A. Crohn's disease.
B. Ulcerative colitis.
C. Leukoplakia.
D. Retinitis Pigmentosa.

Ans: (D)

Precancerous condition

1. Chronic gastritis of Pernicious Anemia.
2. Solar Keratosis of the skin.
3. Chronic ulcerative collitis.
4. Leukoplakia of the oral cavity. Vulva & Penis.
5. Crohn's disease

All these conditions are called precancerous conditions.

Note:

Malignant potential is seen in both ulcerative colitis & Crohn's disease but ulcerative collitis is more important risk factor than Crohn's disease. Diverticular disease and Ischemic collitis *do not predispose to cancer*.

Retinitis Pigmentosa: This primary Pigmentary retinal dystrophy is a hereditary discloser predominantly effecting the rods more than the cones. Most common mode is Autosomal Recessive. It is not a *premalignant condition*.
(Reference: Robinson Page No. 287 7th Edition)

Q.7. Bence John's protein is:

A. Polyclonal Heavy chain
B. Polyclonal Light Chain
C. Monoclonal light chain
D. Monoclonal Heavy Chain

Ans: (C)

Bence jones protein is seen in *Multiple myeloma..* In 99% of patient of Multiple myeloma, electrophoresis reveals level of Ig in blood or monoclonal light chains. Serum M protein & Bence Jones proteinuria are observed in to 70% pts.

Note: Serum *M Protein* is not due to *IgM* but due to *IgG immunoglobulins.*

Q.8. True about natural killer cells are all *except*:

A. Kill Virus
B. Large granular lymphocytes
C. Have azeurophilic granules
D. Mediates Type IV Hypersensitivity

Ans: (D)

1. Nk cells are also called as *large granular Lymphocytes.*
2. Contain *azeurophillic* granules.
3. 1st line defence against Neoplastic cells & virus Laden cells.
4. Not mediated by an Immune response & antigen - antibody reaction.
5. NK cells Express *CD16 & CD 56.*

Q.9. Adult polycystic kidney disease is:

A. Autosomal dominant
B. Autosomal Recessive
C. X-Linked recessive
D. X-Linked dominant

Ans: (A)

A list of Autosomal dominant disease

Adult polycystic disease
Acute Intermittent porphyria
Alzheimer's disease
Alpha-1 Antitrypsin deficiency
Adenomatosis Polyp (Familial)
Huntington's chorea
Marfan syndrome

Many enzyme deficiency diseases are Autosomal recessive.

Like:

Gaucher's disease, Glycogen storage disease, Hurler's & Hunter's disease, sickle cell disease, Tay-sach's disease-phenylketonuria, Albinism, Galactosaemia.

PATHOLOGY

Q.10. Tuberculosis ulcer edges are:

A. Rolled edge.
B. Everted edges.
C. Undermined edges.
D. Punched out edge.

Ans: (C)

Ulcer types	*Edges*
• Non specific ulcer	• Shelving
• Tuberculosis ulcer	• Undermined edges
• Basal-cell carcinoma. (Rodent ulcer)	• Rolled edge
• Epithelioma	• Everted edge
• Syphilis	• Punched out edge

What to do friends, we have to remember always the many lists.

Q.11. What type of Hypersensitivity seen in SLE?

A. Type I hypersensitivity
B. Type II hypersensitivity
C. Type III hypersensitivity
D. Type IV hypersensitivity

Ans: (C)

Try to Remember

Type-I: Immediate Hypersensitivity (Ig E mediated)
Eg: Atopic, Asthma, Hay fever, Anaphylaxis

Type-II: Cytotoxic (Ig G /Ig M Mediated)
Eg: Good Pasture syndrome,Graves disease, Myasthenia gravis, auto-immune hemolytic anemia
Erythroblastosis fetalis.

Type-III: Immune Complexes (IgA/IgG)
Eg:- Arthus reaction, Serum sickness, Rheumatic fever, Glomerulonephritis, SLE

Type-IV: Cell Mediated (delayed) (T cell / macrophages)
Eg: Tuberculosis, Contact dermatitis, Transplant rejection

(Reference: Robbins Page No. 196 16th Edition)

Q.12. Lung carcinoma with worst prognosis:

A. Squamous cell carcinoma

B. Adenocarcinoma

C. Small cell carcinoma

D. Large cell carcinoma

Ans: (C)

Small cell Carcinoma are Highly Malignant and Blood metastasis occurs early.

Try to Remember

M/c variety of lung Carcinoma in India→ **Squamous cell carcinoma.**

M/c variety in world→**Adenocarcinoma**

M/c variety in young patients→ **Adeno-carcinoma**

Carcinoma which metastasis to opposite lung→ **Adenocarcinoma**

Histological variety that cavitates→**Squamous cell carcinoma.**

Lung carcinoma with worst prognosis→**Small cell carcinoma.**

Variety most responsive to chemotherapy & Radiotherapy → **Small cell carcinoma.**

M/c variety with cushing syndrome →**Small cell carcinoma.**

Variety with best prognosis→**Squamous cell carcinoma.**

Variety with central in location→**Squamous cell Carcinoma & Small cell carcinoma.**

Gynaecomastia is seen in which type of carcinoma→**Large cell carcinoma.**

Q.13. Epithelioid Granuloma consists mainly of:

A. Lymphocytes

B. Neutrophills

C. Histiocyte's

D. Macrophages

Ans. (D)

When a persistent antigen present the macro-phages undergo morphologic transformation into epithelium like cells, known as **epitheliod cells.** The **Epitheliod cells** are surrounded by

PATHOLOGY

Lymphocytes, referred as Granuloma, this pattern of inflammation Type-IV Hypersensitivity.

Q.14. All are seen in acute inflammation *except*:

A. Granuloma
B. Increased vascular permeability
C. Vasodilation
D. Neutrophill migration

Ans: (A)

Granuloma formation is seen in chronic inflammatory disease.

Try to Remember

- Histamine increase the vascular permeability and the richest source is Mast cells.
- Serotonin also increase the vascular permeability. The sources are platelet and Enterochromaffin cells.
- Bradykinin is the potent agents, which increases the vascular permeability.
- C3a, C5a and leukotriene C4, D4, E4 Increases the vascular permeability.

Q.15. About Hemolytic anemia all are true *except*:

A. Increased Haptoglobin
B. Reticulocytosis
C. Spherocytes are seen
D. Increased unconjugated bilirubin

Ans: (A)

There is decreased level of Haptoglobins in Hemolytic Anemia. Haptoglobin is a globulin produced by the liver, which binds free Haemoglobin to form a complex not to be excreted by the kidney.

Other feature of Haemolysis

1. Increased Bilirubin
2. Increased LDH (Due to Red cell destruction)
3. Increased Reticulocytes.
4. +ve urinary Haemosiderin.

Q.16. Invasive Carcinoma differs from Carcinoma in situ by:

A. Pleomorphism.
B. Basement membrane Involvement

PATHOLOGY

C. Both
D. None

Ans: (B)

Any Carcinomas that have not invaded through the basement membrane of the dermo epidermal junction known as carcinoma in situ.
Example: Basal cell carcinoma, Paget's disease.

Q.17. Morphology Report says few neutrophil, with heavy, boggy, red lung. What is the stage of lobar pneumonia?

A. Congestion
B. Red hepatization
C. Gray hepatization
D. Resolution

Ans: (A)

In lobar Pneumonia, 4 stages of inflammatory Response.

- *Congestion predominates in the first 24 hours. Morphology Report says few neutrophil, with heavy, boggy, red lung.*
- *Red Hepatization i.e.*—Massive confluent Exudation with Red cells & Neutrophils.
- *Gray Hepatization i.e*—Fibrino-supprative exudates.
- *Resolution i.e*—consolidated exudates.

Q.18. Major Histocompatibility Complex (MHC) have all the characters *except*:

A. Located at short ARM 6th chromosomes.
B. Responsible for graft rejection
C. Have genes of complements.
D. Class II for all nucleated cells.

Ans: (D)

MHC also known as HLA (Human Leukocyte antigen).

Genes codes for Histocompatibility is located short arm of 6th Chromosome.

There are **3 type of HLA**

HLA—**class I**→for all **nucleated cells and platelets**. (HLA -A, HLA-B, HLA-C), **For CD8**

HLA—**Class -II**→expression on **Macrophages,** B cells, T-cells. [HLA-D], **For CD4**
HLA—**Class -III**→**Complement,** TNF α,TNF β.

Q.19. Transplant hyper acute rejection is takes place at most is:
A. Within Few Minutes to hour
B. 1-2 weeks later operation
C. 6 Months later operation
D. After several years

Ans: (A)

- Hyper acute Rejection occurs when performed Antidonar antibodies are present in the circulation of recipient.
- It presents within minutes or hours after transplantation.
- Some times may be recognized. By Surgeon as it rapidly becomes cyanotic mottled and flaccid and may excrete few drops of bloody urine.
- It is a type II hypersensitivity reaction.

Acute rejection: Appears within days. Both Cellular and humoral immunity Play role.

Acute cellular rejection: is most commonly seen within initial months after transplantation.

Q.20. MHC is important in pathogeneses of:
A. Immuno deficiency disease
B. Auto-immune disease
C. Genetic disorder
D. None of the above

Ans. (B)

Class-I Antigen

- Are expressed on all nucleated cells and platelets.
- Encode cell surface glycoprotein.
- They are encoded by three closely relate LOCI HLA-A, HLA-B, HLA-C.
- CD8+ T cells widely express Class-I HLA antigen.

Class-II Antigen

- Are expressed on macrophages, B cells and T cells.
- Encode cell surface Glycoproteins.

Class-III Antigen

- These encodes complements of the Complement system.
- MCH is important in pathogenesis of Autoimmunity. E.g. Strong association has been found between ankylosing spondylitis and HLA B.27, Rheumatoid arthritis and HLA DR4 and many **auto-immune condition** with HLA-DR3.

Important: Several gene code for MHC, the most important one is **Chromosome 6.**

SEVEN

Pharmacology

Q.1. Nicotinic receptors are seen in all *except*:

A. Adrenal medulla
B. Bronchial smooth muscle
C. Skeletal muscle and plate
D. Autonomic ganglia

Ans: (B)

Nicotinic receptors are mainly 2 types

Nm and **Nn**

Nm–are situated in skeletal muscle and plate.

Nn:

- Present on ganglionic cells (sympathetic and parasympathetic)
- Adrenal medullary cells
- Spinal cords
- Certain areas of brain.

Q.2. Disulfiram like reaction is caused by all *except*:

A. Griseofulvin
B. Metronidazole
C. Cephalosporin
D. Erythromycin

Ans: (D)

Drugs causing disulfiram like reaction

Mnemonics:

FMG (Foreign medical graduate) On Competition

F – Furazolidone.
M – Metronidazole.
G – Griseofulvin.
O – Oral hypoglycemics.
C – Cephalosporin.

Q.3. Which of the following is not an anti pseudomonal agent?

A. Vancomycin
B. Ticarcillin
C. Ceftazidime
D. Tobramycin

Ans: (A)

Vancomycin is a glycopeptide antibiotic. It is bactericidal to gram +ve cocci such as Neisseria, clostridia and diphteroids.

It does not act on gram -ve bacilli such as pseudomonas.

It is the drug of choice for

A. Antibiotic associated with **Peudomembranous colitis**

B. **MRSA** (Methicillin resistant staph.aureus)

Its side effects have been asked

- Ototoxic
- Nephrotoxic
- Redman syndrome

Q.4. Heparin Induced thrombocytopenia Tackle by all *except*:

A. Switch on to warfarin
B. Cannot be substituted with LMWH (Low Molecular Weight Heparin)
C. Stop heparin
D. None of the above

Ans: (D)

(Reference: Tripathi 5th Ed. Page No. 562)

Thrombocytopenia is common problem. Generally it is mild and transient occurs due to aggregation of platelets occasionally antibodies are formed to heparin - platelet complex and marked depletion of platelet occurs. So heparin should be discontinued, Even LMW heparins are not safe in such patients.

In *lippincot's* it is written that if heparin induced thrombocytopenia occurs you should give the drug that inhibits platelet aggregation or an oral anticoagulant in place of the heparin.

Some other important points:

- Heparin is a mucopolysaccharide.
- Heparin & insulin does not cross placental barrier, so they are safe in pregnancy.
- Antidote for heparin-Protamine sulphate, whereas antidote for Warfarin-Vit. K.
- M.O.A of heparin-It blocks the action of factor X & thrombin.

Q.5. Prokinetic drug with no dopamine antagonism:

A. Metoclopramide
B. Domperidone
C. Mosapride
D. Chloropromazine

Ans: (C)

(Reference: Tripathi 5th Ed. Page No. 604)

Mosapride acts as 5 HT4 agonist and 5 HT3 antagonist.

It does not produce extrapyramidal, hyperprolactinemic side effects due to absence of D2 blocking property.

All other drugs mentioned in the option block the D2 receptors.

Prokinetic Drugs—These are drugs which promote gastrointestinal transit & gastric emptying.

ONDANSETRON - It is 5-HT antagonists. It is used to control cancer chemotherapy/ radiotherapy induced vomiting.

Q.6. Drug which does not interfere with antacid:

A. Azithromycin
B. Tetracycline
C. Norfloxacin
D. Ranitidine

Ans : (A)

(Reference: Tripathi 5th Ed. Page No. 596)

Drug interactions of antacid:

By raising gastric PH & by forming complexes the nonabsorbable antacids decreases the absorption of many drugs specially tetracycline,

Iron salts, Fluoroquinolones (Ciprofloxacin, Norfloxacin) H2 blockers, Ketoconazole, Phenytoin, Isoniazid, Ethambutol and Nitrofurantoin.

Macrolides are not mentioned in drug interaction of antacid.

Q.7. Not used as an antacid:

A. $NaHCo_3$

B. $Al\,OH_3$

C. $CaCO_3$

D. $MgSo_4$

Ans: (D)

(Reference: Tripathi 5 Ed. Page No. 595)

$MgSo_4$ is not used as an antacid but Magnesium Hydroxide and Magnesium Trisillicate are used as an Antacid

$MgSo_4$ is the Drug of choice in Eclampsia as anticonvulsant

Q.8. β Blockers are used in all *except*:

A. A-V Block

B. Angina

C. Familial tremor

D. Cardiac Arrythmias

Ans: (A)

(Reference: Tripathi 5th Ed Page No. 129)

Please remember the indication of propranolol and side effect of Phenytoin. In every exam these 2 drugs are asked.

Use of Propanol

Mnemonic **-THAPAD**

T - **T**hyrotoxicosis

H - **H**ypertension

A - **A**nxiety

P - **P**heochromocytoma

A - **A**ngina

D - **D**igitalis Toxicity

*Migraine (for chronic prophylaxis)

*Essential tremor of thyrotoxicosis

*Familial Tremor

Toxicity of Phenytoin

Pneumonic - GAVE GAS For Life

G – Gum Hyperplasia
A – Ataxia
V – Vision Blurred
E – Enlarged liver
GAS – **GA**Stric upset
For – Folate deficiency
Life – Lymphoma like syndrome

Q.9. All are Beta lactam inhibitors *except:*

A. Astreonam
B. Sulbactam
C. Tazobactam
D. Clavulanic Acid

Ans: (A)

(Reference: Tripathi 5th Ed. Page No. 662)

Beta Lactam inhibitors are

1. Clavulanic acid
2. Sulbactam
3. Tazobactam.

Q.10. Warfarin acts by inhibiting which factors:

A. XII
B. VIII
C. VII
D. III

Ans: (C)

(Reference: K. D. Tripathi 5th Ed. Page No. 564)

Warfarin act indirectly by Interfering with the synthesis of vit.K dependent clotting factors in liver. They apparently behave as competitive antagonists of vit.K and reduce plasma levels of functional clotting factors in a dose dependent manner.

Vit.K dependent factors are 10, 9, 7, 2.

The dose of oral anticoagulant must be individualized by repeated measurement of Prothrombin time.

Important Point:

- Antidote for heparin is **protamine sulfate.**
- The anticoagulant action of heparin is exerted mainly by Inhibition of factor Xa as well as thrombin IIa mediated conversion of fibrinogen to fibrin.

Q.11. Warfarin metabolism is inhibited by:

A. Cimetidine
B. Rifampin
C. Griseofulvin
D. Indometacin

Ans: (A)

(Reference: Tripathi 5th Ed. Page No. 567)

Drugs which inhibit **warfarin metabolism** are:

- Chloramphenicol
- Erythromycin
- Celecoxib
- Cimentidine
- Allopurinol
- Amiodarone
- Metronidazole

*Drugs which displace **warfarin from plasma protein** are:*

- Sulfonamides
- Indometacin
- Probenacid

*Drugs which induce the **metabolism of oral anticoagulant** are:*

- Rifampin
- Griseofulvin.

Q.12. Anti TB Drug causing Gout:

A. Pyrazinamide
B. Streptomycin
C. Isoniazid
D. Rifampicin

Ans: (A)

(Reference: Harrison 15th Ed. Page No. 1019)

S/E of Antitubercular drugs:

Hyperuricaemia
- Ethambutol
- Pyrazinamide

Peripheral neuropathy
- Streptomycin
- INH
- Ethambutol
- Ethionamide

Hepatitis
- Isoniazid
- Rifampicin
- Pyrazinamide

Optic Neuritis
- Isoniazid
- Ethambutol

Ototoxicity & renal toxicity →Streptomycin
Pigmentation →Rifampicin
Thiacetazone is contraindicated in HIV patient because causes **EXFOLIATIVE DERMATITIS.**

Q.13. In a patient with hepatitis which ATT is most safe:

A. S+E
B. H+E
C. R+E
D. S+H

Ans: (A)

Antitubercular drugs which causes hepatitis are:
Isoniazid (H)
Rifampicin (R)
Pyrazinamide (Z)
So **Ethambutol(E)** and **Streptomycin(S)** does not cause hepatitis. So they are safe in patient with hepatitis.

Q.14. Pancreatitis is a S/E of:

A. Didanosine
B. Tenofovir
C. Zidovudine
D. Saquinavir

Ans: (A)

(Reference: Harrison 16th Ed. Page No. 1125)

Didanosine

It is best absorbed on empty stomach at high PH. The most common toxicity is painful sensory peripheral neuropathy. Didanosine is contraindicated in patient with a prior history of pancreatitis, regardless of etiology.

Zalcitabine also cause pancreatitis.

Lamivudine is among the best tolerated with least toxic nucleoside analogue.

S/E of zidovudine are *macrocytic anemia, çardiomyopathy & Lactic acidosis*.

Tenofovir - S/E- Renal toxicity

Antiretroviral drugs which do not cause peripheral neuropathy

1. Lamivudine
2. Zidovudine

Antiretroviral drugs causing peripheral neuropathy

1. Zalcitabine
2. Didanosine
3. *Stamivudine*

Q.15. Lactic Acidosis is most commonly caused by which oral hypoglycemic drug:

A. Phenformin
B. Metformin
C. Tolbutamide
D. Glipizide

Ans: (A)

(Reference: K.D. 5th Ed. Page No. 247)

Lactic acidosis is caused by both phenformin and metformin.

But lactic acidosis m/c caused by phenformin.

Q.16. Drug of Choice in LGV:

A. Tetracycline
B. Doxycycline
C. Erythromycin
D. Ampicillin

Ans: (B)

(Reference: K.D. Tripathi 5th Ed. Page No. 696)

May be you are thinking that Doc is tetracycline. But in KDT 5th Ed Page No. 696. Tetracycline is not mentioned in the treatment of STD's.

The Ist choice of drugs are :

- Azithromycin 1g of single dose orally.
- Doxycycline 100 mg BD X 7 days.

Some other tricky questions:

DOC for cholera treatment is - **Doxycyline**

DOC for the prophylaxis of cholera - **Tetracycline**

Doxycycline is contraindicated in Pregnancy. So **FURAZOLIDONE** is the Antibiotic of choice for pregnant woman in cholera.

TMP-SMX is the antibiotic of choice for children. **Tetracycline** is equally effective but is not available everywhere in paediatric form.

Plague

The DOC for plague is - **streptomycin**

The DOC for the prophylaxis of plague is - **Tetracycline.**

Migraine

Sumatriptan is the DOC in the treatment of acute migraine.

Propranolol is effective for prophylaxis of migraine.

Q.17. All of the following can cause haemolytic anemia in G-6PD deficiency, *except:*

A. Primaquine

B. Sulphonamide

C. Penicillin

D. Aspirin in large dosage

Ans: (C)

This is a very frequently asking question.

Remember:

Drugs causing hemolysis in G6PD "Deficiency"

Mnemonics:

Did **SAN**i**A** **C**ompetitive **P**layer.

D - *Dapsone*

S - *Sulfonamide*

A - *Antimalarials e.g. Primaquine*

N - *Nitrofurantoin , Nalidixic acid*

A - *Aspirine, Aminosalicylic acid*

C - *Cotrimoxazole, Chloramphenicol*

P - *Phenacetin , Probenecid , Procainamide.*

(Reference: Page No. 433, Harrison, 15th Edition).

Q.18. Newer type of retinoids are:

A. Adapalene
B. Tretinoin
C. Casipotriel
D. Azelaic acid

Ans: (A)

Adapalene: It is the **Newer Synthetic Tretinoin** like drug which binds directly to the **Nuclear Retinoic Acid Receptor** and modulates Keratinization and Differentiation of **Follicular Epithelial cells.** It also exert **Anti inflammatory action.** In Acne vulgaris it is effective.

(Reference: Page No: 801, K.D.Tripathi.)

EIGHT

Anaesthesiology

Q.1. Pin Index of oxygen is:

A. 0.5
B. 1.5
C. 2.5
D. 3.5

Ans: (C)

Pin Index system

This is safety mechanism so that one cylinder cannot be fitted at other's position. The pins are so positioned that one cylinder with corresponding hole can only be fitted.

Some imp. Pin index.

- Oxygen —**2.5**
- Nitrous Oxide—**3.5**
- Cyclopropane—**3.6**
- Air—**1.5**
- Nitrogen—**1.4**
- Entonox (50% 02 + 50% nitrous oxide) —**7**
- Carbon dioxide (<7.5%)—**2.6**
- Carbondioxide (.7.5%)—**1.6**

(Reference: Yadav, Page No.21,2nd Edition)

Q.2. Anaesthesia agent with least analgesic property:

A. N_2O
B. Halothane
C. Ethers
D. Propane

Ans: (B)

Halothane is a potent anaesthetic but poor analgesic.

Remember

- Maximum Analgesic—Trilene
- Profound Analgesic —Ketamine
- Only Analgesic —N2O
- Analgesic—Halothane

Remember

- Post spinal headache starts in 1st 3 days and last for 1-2 weeks. Most painful on IV injection -propofal
- Gag reflex is through - 9th cranial nerve.
- Atracurium is metabolized by Hoffmann degradation.
- Suxamethonium is metabolized in plasma by pseudocholine esterase.
- Suxamethonium increase intra cranial pressure & intra ocular tension.

Q.3. Used for IV Induction *except*:

A. Thiopentone Na
B. Ketamine
C. Etomidate
D. Bupivacine

Ans: (D)

Commonly used IV induction

Thiopentone
Propafol
Ketamine
Etomidate
Midazolum
Althesin
Methohexirone

Some important points

- IV Anaesthesia of choice in **day care surgery is—propofol**
- Sodium Thiopentone is ultra short acting due to— **rapid redistribution**
- Dissociative anaesthesia is seen in— **Ketamine**
- Post spinal headache is due to—**CSF Leak**

- Conc. of lidocaine used in spinal anaesthesia **•5%**

Lignocaine use in different concentration:

5% Spinal anaesthesia

4% Topically in eye

0.5% Epidural anesthesia

Q.4. Spinal Anesthesia should be injected into the space between:

A. T_{12} -L_1

B. L_3 -L_4

C. L_1 - L_2

D. L_5-S_1

Ans: (B)

- The LA is injected in the sub arachnoid space between L_2-L_3 or L_3-L_4.
- Spinal cord extends from medulla oblongata to lower border of L_1 in adult.
- Spinal cord extends from medulla oblongata to lower border of L_3 in infant & neonate. (adult level achieved at 2 years of age)
- In infancy spinal anesthesia given at L_4-L_5 level.
- In adult spinal anesthesia given at L_3-L_4 OR L_4-L_5 space. (even at L_2-L_3)
- In adult usually spinal anesthesia given at L_3-L_4 level.

Remember: structures *encountered during spinal anesthesia*

1-skin, **2**-subcutaneous tissue, **3**-supraspinous ligament, **4**-Interspinous ligament, **5**-ligament flavum, **6**-dura, 7-arachnoid.

(Reference: Yadav, Page No. 116 and 117,2nd Edition)

Q.5. Laughing gas is:

A. Nitrous oxide

B. Halothane

C. Cyclopropane

D. Entonox.

ANAESTHESIOLOGY

Ans: (A)

Remember

- Laughing gas—**Nitrous oxide, name given by Humphry dary.**
- Vomiting gas —**Chloropicrin.**
- Tear gas—**Aceton, benzene bromide & xylol.**
- Suffocating gas—**chlorine, phosgen, oxychlorocarban.**
- Sneezing gas—**diphenylchlorasine.**
- Noble gas—**helium, neon, argon, krypton, xenon, radon.**

(Reference: Stedman's Medical Dictionary)

NINE

Orthopaedics

Q.1. In carpel tunnel syndrome the nerve involved is:

A. Auxillary nerve
B. Radial nerve
C. Ulnar nerve
D. Median nerve

Ans: (D)

- The median nerve is compressed in the carpel tunnel syndrome
- The ulnar nerve is compressed in the cubital tunnel syndrome
- The tibial nerve is compressed in the tarsal tunnel syndrome

The cause of "Carpel tunnel syndrome"

Mnemonics *GRAMPIT*

G —Gout
R —Rheumatoid arthritis
A —Acromegaly
M—Myxoedema
P —Pregnancy
I —Idiopathic
T —Trauma

Diagnosed by: *Electromyography and nerve conduction studies.*

Q.2. Fibrous ankylosis is seen in:

A. Septic arthritis
B. TB arthritis
C. Psoriatic arthritis
D. Bechet's disease

Ans: (B)

Ankylosis is 2 types:

1. Fibrous ankylosis→Healing by fibrosis, limitation or near complete loss of joint movement is known as fibrous ankylosis.
2. Bony ankylosis → Destruction of articular cartilage has occurs at the joint space is completely lost and traversed by bony trabecular between the bones forming the joint.

Fibrous ankylosis is the outcome of healed tuberculosis except in spine where bony ankylosis occurs.

Q.3. Metacarpophalangeal joints are most common affected in:

A. Osteoarthritis
B. Psoriasis
C. Rheumatic Arthritis
D. Pseudo gout

Ans: (C)

Rheumatoid arthritis: Metacarpophalangeal (MCP) Joint especially of index finger, proximal interphalangeal joint, wrist, elbow, knee, ankle. Distal interphalangeal is not involved characteristically.

Osteoarthritis: Joint involved Proximal interphalangeal, Distal interphalangeal, base of thumb

Sparing of wrist and metacarpophalangeal joint.

Psoriasis: Joint involved Proximal interphalangeal, Distal interphalangeal wrist, Metacarpophalangeal joint.

Q.4. Hill – Sach's lesion seen in:

A. Anterior dislocation of hip
B. Posterior dislocation of hip
C. Recurrent dislocation of shoulder
D. Posterior dislocation of shoulder

Ans: (C)

Hill Sach's lesion and Bankart's lesion causes recurrent dislocation of shoulder.

In previous year they asked about the Luxation

in erecta which is also known as downward/ Inferior dislocation.

Most common Type of Shoulder dislocation → anterior dislocation of shoulder (sub-coracoid type) dislocation.

Surgeries for Recurrent dislocation of shoulder:
- Bankart's operation
- Puti platt's operation
- Bristow's operation.

Q.5. Nerve damaged in the shaft of humerus fracture:

A. Median nerve
B. Radial nerve
C. Ulnar nerve
D. Axillary nerve

Ans: (B)

Most common nerve involved in:
- Anterior dislocation of shoulder–*Axillary nerve*
- #Surgical neck of Humerus–*Axillary nerve*
- #Shaft of Humerus–*Radial nerve*
- #Supracondylar Humerus—*Median nerve*
- Volkman's ischemic contracture–*Median nerve*
- *Dislocation of lunate–Median nerve.*

Q.6. Tinel's sign is seen in:

A. Regeneration
B. Degeneration
C. Both
D. None

Ans: (A)

Tinel's Sign:

On gently taping over the course of the nerve from distal to proximal, a sensation of current or hyperesthesia is felt in skin which supplied by the involved nerve.

Tinel's sign and motor examination is the sign of regeneration.

Motor Examination:

The muscle supplied nearest to the site of injury is 1st to recover. It is also known as *MOTOR MARCH*.

Types of nerve injury:

- Neuropraxia "it is the compression of any nerve, in which physiological function is lost but anatomical nerve is intact".
- Axonotemesis "in which some of the axon are injured, but nerve is intact".
- Neurotemesis "in which the nerve is not intact, here nerve is totally injured. So regeneration of the nerve is very poor".

Neuroma: if any muscle tissue or any fibrous is takes place in between the proximal and distal stamp of nerve injury site, then Axonal sprouting from proximal stamp unable to go distal stamp. So also sprouted axons will make formation of **neuroma,** which is also known as *Traumatic Neuroma*. **Tinel's sign** is +ve because of neuroma formation.

TEN

Radiology

Q.1. Most radiosensitive tissue of the body is:

A. Bone marrow
B. Nervous Tissue
C. Connective Tissue
D. Fat Tissue

Ans: **(A)**

Remember

- Least Radiosensitive Tissue of body—nervous tissue
- Least Radio sensitive blood cell—Platelet
- Most radio sensitive blood cell—Lymphocyte
- Most radio resistant organ—Vagina
- Most common organ to be affected by radiation—Skin

Q.2. Double bubble sign in Barium meal seen in:

A. Duodenal Atresia
B. Jejunal Atresia
C. Ileocaecal kochs
D. Ulcerative colitis

Ans: (A)

Single bubble appearance is seen in—**Pyloric stenosis.**

Double bubble appearance is seen in —**Duodenal Artesia, Annular pancreas.**

Triple Bubble appearance is seen in—**Jejunal Artesia**

Multiple air fluid levels are seen in—**Intestinal obstruction.**

Gas under diaphragm seen in— **Pneumoperitoneum**

RADIOLOGY

Q.3. Element M/C used in Brachytheraphy of Carcinoma cervix:

A. Radium-226
B. Cobalt-60
C. Gold-198
D. Caesiom-137

Ans: (D)

Brachytheraphy: Type of radiation in which radioactive sources are placed in dose proximity to or directly into tumors.

Intestial

RT Needles Placed into Prostate/penis/other soft tissue.)

Intracavitary

eg. In urethra (m/c used **cs137**)

M/C used source in Brachytherapy - Ir190. C.S.I.

REMEMBER, some commonly asked half life of ISOTOPES

- ***Radium 226——1620 years***
- ***Caesium- 137—30 years***
- ***Cobalt 60——5.3 years***
- ***Iridium 192—74.4 years***
- ***Iodine 125——60 days***
- ***Phosphorus32—14.3 days***
- ***Gold 198—2.7 days***

RADIOLOGY

Q.4. Filament in X-ray made of:

A. Tungsten filament
B. Chromium
C. Gallium
D. Selenium

Ans: (A)

Please remember: *Target is not Tungsten in mammography, its made up off molybdenum.*

Q.5. Investigation of choice in a person brought with traumatic paraplegia is:

A. MRI
B. CT
C. Myelography
D. USG

Ans: (A)

- All spinal imaging is done by MRI
- MRI is safe in pregnancy

Unit of MRI is TESLA.

Q.6. Best method to diagnose pathology in terminal part of CBD by:

A. USG
B. ERCP
C. PTC
D. CECT

Ans: (B)

Under radiological control the ampula of vater is cannulated and the common bile duct or pancreatic duct can be entered .Contrast medium can then be injected and the biliary or pancreatic duct can be shown. It is method of choice for the investigation of **obstructive jaundice**. It is also of great value in the investigation of **pancreatic disease.**

ELEVEN

Psychiatry

Q.1. Drug of choice in depression in old person is:

A. Fluoxetine
B. Buspirone
C. Amitryptyline
D. Imipramine

Ans: (A)

Fluoxetine is devoid of anticholinergic, hypotensive and sedative side effects, so safer with cardiac disease and BPH.

Q.2. DOC in OCD

A. Sertraline
B. Alprazom
C. Chlorpromazine
D. Clomipramine

Ans: (D)

Other important Points

- DOC for Attention Deficit Hyperactive Disorder—Methyl phenidate
- DOC for delirium tremens—diazepam
- Resistant case of schizophrenia—clozapine
- DOC for Gillesla Tourette's syndrome—Haloporidol
- TOC for depression with suicidal tendency—ECT (electro convulsive therapy)
- DOC for treatment of manic episode is—Lithium
- DOC in Nocturnal Enuresis—Imipramine
- DOC in Rapid cycling bipolar disorder—Na-valproate

(Reference: Batra, Page No. 88 1st Edition, Ahuja Page No. 100, 5th Ed)

Q.3. Prophylactic maintenance serum level of lithium is:

A. 0.2-0.8 mEq/l
B. 0.7-1.2 mEq/l
C. 1.2-2.0 mEq/l
D. 2.0-2.5 mEq/l

Ans: (B)

Dose of Lithium should be remembered

- *Therapeutic* level dose - 0.8-1.2 mEq/ l—for Rx. of acute mania.
- *Prophylactic* level - 0.6-1.2 mEq/——for Rx. of relapse prevention in bipolar disorder.
  - *Toxic level* - >2 mEq/ l
  - *Life threatening intoxication*—3.5mEq/ l

(Reference: Ahuja, Page No. 196,5th Edition)

Q.4. False perception without external stimulus is:

A. Illusion
B. Hallucination
C. Delirium
D. Delusion

Ans: (B)

Remember these definitions they are important

- **Illusion**—Is misinterpretation of stimuli arising from external object
- **Delusion**—Is a false unshakable belief, which is not amenable to reasoning and is in keeping the patient with socio-cultural and educational background.
  In short—**false but firm** belief.
- **Delirium**—Is an acute confusion state characterized by alteration in consciousness orientation and perception.

(Reference: Ahuja, Page No. 14,5th Edition)

TWELVE

Skin and STD

Q.1. Latest retinoid drug used in psoriasis:

A. Adapalene
B. Tretnoin
C. Calcipotriol
D. Tazarotene

Ans: (D)

– Tazarotene-vitamin-A agonist (retinoid) has also come into clinical use recently. It tends not to induce clearance and may cause irritation.

– Calcipotriol-It is a vit.D agonist. It tends to reduce the thickness of the plaque and diminish the scaring.

Acne vulgaris use of retinoid -*DAVIDSON 19th Ed. Page No. 1082.*

Studies of use of topical andsystemic retinoid in Acne vulgaris have shown that:

1. Adapalene is more rapid in onset andbetter tolerated than tretnoin in mild to moderate acne.
2. Oral isotretnoin is clinically better and more cost effective in moderate and severe acne. *So adapalene-retinoid drug used in acne not in psoriasis.*

(Reference: Davidson 19th Edition Page NO. 1078)

Q.2. Alopecia, Hyper pigmentation, Hypogonadism characteristic for deficiency of

A. Zinc
B. Magnesium
C. Selenium
D. Copper

Ans: (A)

The essential feature of Zinc deficiency:

1. A distinctive rash most often around the eyes, nose, mouth, anus and distal parts called **Acrodermatitis Enteropathica**.
2. Growth retardation in children.
3. Impaired wound healing.
4. Hypogonadism with diminished reproductive capacity.
5. Anorexia often accompanied by diarrhoea
6. Depressed mental function.

Other important disease

Selenium deficiency causes Keshan disease.

Copper deficiency causes Menke's disease.

(Reference: Robbins 7th Edition Page No. 1161)

Q.3. Isomorphism not seen in:

A. Lichen planus

B. Warts

C. Psoriasis

D. Vitiligo

Ans: (D)

Isomorphism or Koebner phenomenon-It means linear lesions produced by scratching a primary lesion which results in new lesions developing along the line of the scratch. *Eg*: Lichen planus,warts and psoriasis. But ***koebner phenomenon*** is characteristic for *Lichen planus*.

(Reference: Dermatology P.N.Behl, Page No. 31)

Q.4. Decrease number of melanocyte is seen in:

A. Albinism

B. Piebaldism

C. Ichthyosis

D. Chemical leucoderma

Ans: (B)

Piebaldism is a Autosomal dominant disease characterised by patches of skin that lack melanin as a result of defect in migration of melanoblasts from neural crest to skin.

Skin biopsy: Hypomelanotic area-few to no melanocytes.

Vitiligo: is an acquired disease and similar patch of loss of melanin, but the loss develops after birth and progressive.

Albinism: Congenital inability to synthesize melanin.

(Reference: Harrison 16th Edition. Page No. 301)

Q.5. Not a cutaneous manifestation of TB:

A. Lupus pernio
B. Lupus vulgaris
C. Erythema nodosum
D. Scrofuloderma

Ans: (A)

Lupus pernio is a skin manifestation of Sarcoidosis.

- Sarcoidosis does not involve kidney.
- Sarcoidosis mimics like Berylliosis.

THIRTEEN

ENT

Q1. External Ear is not supplied by which nerve:

A. Greater auricular nerve
B. Lesser occipital nerve
C. Auriculo temporal nerve
D. Glossopharyngeal nerve

Ans: (D)

External Ear is supplied by greater auricular (C-2,3), lesser occipital (C2), auricular branch of vagus, auriculo temporal nerve - mandibular division, some fibers of facial nerve.

Auriculo temporal nerve supply:

Anterior wall, roof of meatus and anterior part of tympanic membrane

Vagus nerve supply:

Posterior wall, floor of meatus and posterior part of tympanic membrane.

Tympanic plexus supply:

Medial side of tympanic membrane.

(Reference: P.L. Dhingra-5th Page)

Q.2. Tonsils are innervated by which nerve:

A. Vagus
B. Glossopharyngeal
C. Abducent nerve
D. Facial nerve

Ans: (B)

Tonsil (palatine tonsil)

Innervated by - sphenopalatine ganglion (v) and glossopharyngeal nerve.

Blood supply - Five arteries

1. Tonsilar branch of facial artery **(main artery)**
2. Ascending pharyngeal artery
3. Ascending palatine

4. Dorsal lingual branches
5. Descending palatine artery

Venous drainage - Facial vein and pharyngeal venous plexus.

Q.3. Pure tone is:

A. Multiple frequency
B. Single frequency
C. Frequency above 4000 Hz
D. Frequency less than 4000Hz

Ans: (B)

Pure tone: *Single frequency sound is called a pure tone from 125 to 8000 Hz.*

Complex sound: *Sound with more than one frequency of sound.*

Try to remember this

Whisper: **30 dB**

Normal conversation: **60 dB**

Shout: **90 dB**

Discomfort of the ear: **120 dB**

(Reference: P. No. 23, P.L. Dhingra)

Q.4. Schwartz sign is seen in:

A. Schwannoma
B. Otosclerosis
C. Glomus tumour
D. Facial nerve palsy

Ans: (B)

Schwartz sign: Flamingo: pink blue may be seen on tymphanic membrane due to increased vascularity, this is pathognomic feature of otosclerosis.

Otosclerosis (otospongiosis)

It is primary disease of bony labyninth by characterized by alternating phase of bone resorption and formation.

3 types:

a. Stapedial (M/c)
b. Cochlear
c. Histological.

ENT

Some Important features

1. Schwartz sign
2. Negative Rinne's test
3. Cohortz notch at 2000 Hz.

Rx - *Stapedectomy is the treatment of choice.*

Q.5. Bullous myringitis is caused by:

A. Pseudomonas
B. Streptococci
C. Herpes simplex
D. H. influenza

Ans: (D)

Bullous myringitis caused by virus (H.influenza)
C/F: Haemorrhagic blebs on lateral surface of tymphanic membrane and external auditory canal.
Most common organism responsible for

1. Acute epiglotitis—H. influenza
2. Acute laryngotracheobronchitis (croup)-parainfluenza virus
3. Acute tonsillitis—β-hemolytic streptococcus.
4. *Malignant otitis externa-pseudomonas aeruginosa*

Q.6. In BERA the wave IV orgin from:

A. Cochlear nuclei
B. VIII nerve
C. Lateral leminiscus
D. Medial geniculate body

Ans: (C)

BERA → Auditory brain stem response for non-invasive method to find integrity of central auditory pathway through VIII nerve, pons and mid brain.
In a normal person 7 waves are produced.
1st, 3rd, 5th - most stable waves.
The Anatomic site of orgin of waves as follows:
Wave I—VIIIth nerve
Wave II—Cochlear nuclei (pons)
Wave III—Superior olivary complex (pons)
Wave IV—Lateral leminiscus (pons)
Wave V—Inferior colliculus
Wave VI—Medial geniculate body

Wave VII—Auditory radiations (thalamo-cortical)

Bera used to find threshold hearing in *infants and retrocochlear pathology.*

(Reference: Page No. 32, P.L. Dhingra)

Q.7. About rhinoscleroma false is:

A. Caused by GM +ve bacillus

B. Mikulicz cells

C. Russel bodies

D. Streptomycin is used in treatment

Ans: (A)

Rhinoscleroma is caused by Klebsiella Rhinoscleromatis which is Gr -ve bacillus.

- Starts in nose, extends to nasopharynx, oropharynx, larynx mostly subglottic region.
- In biopsy—plasma cells, lymphocytes, eosinophils, mikulicz cells and russel bodies.
- Mikulicz and russel bodies—diagnostic features.

Rx:

Streptomycin (1g/day) + tetracycline (2g/day) both are given together

(Reference: Page No. 152/ P. L. Dhingra)

ENT

Q.8. Le-Forte's fracture is seen in:

A. Maxilla

B. Mandible

C. Orbital bone

D. Zygomatic arch

Ans: (A)

Fracture of maxilla is divided into 3 types:

Le-Forte I - *Transverse*

Le-Forte II - *Pyramidal*

Le-Forte III - *Craniofacial dysfunction*

Fracture of mandible —Dingman's classification M/c in condylar process of mandibule fracture of orbital floor are called "**Blow out fractures**".

(Reference: Page No. 185 - P.L. Dhingra)

Q.9. Diffuse External Ear Infection are M/c caused by:

A. Virus

B. H. influenza

C. Pseudomonas aeruginosa

D. Actinomyces

Ans: (C)

- Diffuse otitis externa are also known as topical ear or Singapore ear.
- Caused by
  - Pseudomonas aeruginosa (M/c)
  - Bacillus proteus
  - *Staphylococcus Aureus*

  Rx
  - Ear toileting.
  - Antibiotics with steroids.
  - Analgesics.

Q.10. Differential diagnosis between peritonsillar abscess and tonsillitis:

A. Pain

B. Odynophagia

C. Uvula drawn to opposite side

D. Ear ache

Ans: (C)

Pain in throat may be in both quinsy and Tonsillitis

Odynophagia: Difficulty in swallowing may be in both but it is more marked in quinsy.

Ear ache: This is referred pain by a 9th cranial nerve which supply both the tonsil and ear.

In quinsy uvula is swollen and edematous and pushed to opposite side.

Other features of quinsy:

Muffled and thick voice Hot potato voice,

There is marked Odynophagia and Foul breath.

If conservative measure fail to cure Quinsy. Then incision and drainage will be required.

Note: Tonsils are removed **Four to Six** weeks following an attack of Quinsy.

Tonsillitis:

- Most common cause of acute tonsillitis is **Beta Hemolytic strepto cocci.**
- Acute tonsillitis is more common in children but peritonsillar abscess (Quinsy) mostly affects adults. Which are mostly unilateral.
- *Penicillin is the drug of the choice for acute tonsillitis.*

(Reference: Page No. 318, Dhingra, 3rd Edition)

Q.11. Hearing nucleus is:

A. Inferior colliculus

B. Superior calliculus

C. Pons

D. Medulla

Ans: (A)

Remember:

- Midbrain has posteriorly tectum which is made up of left and right, Superior and inferior calliculi.
- Transverse section of midbrain at the level of inferior calliculi the graymatter have Trochlear and Mesencephalic nucleus. Inferior calliculus receives afferent form lateral lemniscus, and gives **efferent's to the Medial geniculate body. In** past, it was considered as the centre for auditory reflexes, the available evidence indicates that it helps in localizing the source of sound.
- The transverse section of midbrain at the level of superior caliculi, the graymatter contains occulomotor and mesencephalic nucleus. The superior colliculus receives afferently from retina and gives efferent to spinal cord.
- **L**ateral geniculate - **L**ight (For Vision)
- **M**edial geniculate - **M**usic (For hearing)

(Reference: Page No: 256, BDC-Volume Third, 3rd Edition)

FOURTEEN

Medicine

Q.1. Post exposure prophylaxis, for HIV patient minimum for:

A. 6 weeks
B. 4 weeks
C. 12 weeks
D. 8 weeks

Ans: (B)

A combination of two **nucleoside reverse transcriptase** inhibitor plus a **protease inhibitors for 4 weeks**.

→ Zidovudine + Lamivudine + Indinavir for 4 weeks.

(Reference: Harrison, 15th Edition, Page No. 1990)

Q.2. Dressler's syndrome is due to:

A. Autoimmune
B. Bacteria
C. Idiopathic
D. Virus

Ans: (A)

Dressler's syndrome is a post myocardial infarction syndrome is characterized by (3P) **Pyrexia, Pancreatitis and Pleurisy** and is probably due to autoimmunity. The syndrome tends to occur a few weeks or even months after the infarct and subsides after a few days. Prolonged or severe symptom may require treatment with high dose Aspirin, a non steroidal anti inflammatory drug or even corticosteroid.

Q.3. Normal Anion gap acidosis seen in:

A. Uremia

B. DKA
C. Lactic Acidosis
D. Cholera

Ans: (D)

Anion gap is increased in:

Mnemonics "KUSSMAUL"

K–**K**etosis with Diabetes, Alcoholism, malnutrition
U–**U**raemia
SS–**S**alicylate Poisoning
M–**M**ethanol Poisoning
U–**U**raemia
L–**L**actic Acidosis

Normal Anion gap is seen in → Diarrhoea and Renal Tubular Acidosis Normal Anion gap in health range from 8 to 14 mmol/ltr.

Q.4. Most common cause of Intracerebral Bleeding is due to:

A. Thrombocytopenia
B. Diabetes
C. Hypertension
D. Berry Aneurysm

Ans: (C)

Remember these points by Heart:

Intracerebral (Parenchymatous Hemorrhage)

- Most common type of Intra cranial Hemorrhage.
- Most common cause is Hypertension causing rapture of small of small perforating arteries or Arterioles.
- Most common site is putamen.

Subarachnoid Hemorrhage

- Most common cause is spontaneous rupture of saccular Aneurysm i.e. Berry Aneurysm.
- Most common site of berry aneurysm is anterior circulation of Willis.

(Reference: Harrison 16th Edition. Page No. 2388)

Q.5. Severity of Mitral stenosis is determined by:

MEDICINE

A. Diastolic murmur Duration
B. Mid D.M
C. Opening Snap
D. Intensity of SI

Ans: (A)

Some important points on Mitral stenosis

- S_1—Accentuated (S1 is soft in calcified heart valve)
- S_2 Normally split S2 with P2 component accentuated
- Murmur—Low pitched rumbling, diastolic murmur heard best at the apex in left lateral recumbent position.
- Opening snap—Brief high pitched, early diastolic sound. It is best heard at the lower left sternal border.

Q.6. 28 years old female presents complaints of tightness of finger and dysphagia. Which of the following is probable diagnosis?

A. Dermatomyositis
B. Scleroderma
C. Rheumatoid Arthritis
D. Polyarteritis Nodosa

Ans: (B)

Diagnosis of this patient is suggested by:

- Evidence of fibrosis of skin
- Evidence of visceral involvement
- Epidemiological characteristic
- Tightness of fingers
- Oesophageal motility or Dysphagia
- Peak incidence of scleroderma is seen in women during the 3rd to 5th decade.

Q.7. 45 years old man complaints of back pain and joint pain in X-ray b/l sacroileitis diagnosis is:

A. Ankylosing spondylitis
B. Psoriatic arthritis
C. RA
D. Scleroderma

Ans: (A)

Important point about Ankylosis spondylitis

It is associated with HLA B-27

Sacroileitis:

- Histologically it is a chronic Synovitis causes **destruction of articular cartilage and bony ankylosis** especially in the sacroiliac joint.
- The onset is usually insidious with recurrent episodes of low back pain and stiffness sometimes radiating to the buttocks or thighs. Characteristically the symptoms are worse in the early morning and after inactivity.
- Some characteristic features of ankylosing spondylitis.
  - Bamboospine
  - Squaring of vertebrae
  - Calcification of IV Disease.
  - Enthesopathy.

Remember

Osteoarthritis

Involvement of PIP, DIP and 1st carpometacarpal joint (base of thumb), sparing of MCP and Wrist.

Rheumatoid Arthritis

Involvement of any small joints of hand i.e.PIP, MCP, Wrist, Sparing of DIP.

Psoriatic arthritis

Involvement of PIP. DIP. MCP and wrist

Sparing of any joint or may not be present.

(Reference: Harrison 16th Edition, Page No. 1214)

Q.8. Morphine is given in:

A. LVF

B. Head Injury

C. Emphysema

D. Cor pulmonale

Ans: (A)

Morphine is given in acute left ventricular failure:

Morphine affords dramatic relief by

- Reducing preload on heart due to vaso-dilatation and peripheral pooling of blood.

MEDICINE

- Tending to shift blood from Pulmonary to systemic circuit relieves pulmonary congestion and edema.
- Cut down sympathetic stimulation by calming the patient reduces cardiac work.

Morphine is contraindicated in

- ICT
- Asthma
- Respiratory Insufficiency, emphysema, Pulmonary fibrosis, corpulmonale
- Head Injury
- Undiagnosed acute abdominal pain

Note: **Treatment of choice in Inferior wall MI/ right ventricular infarction is IV fluids.**

Q.9. Tetany is not seen in:

A. Verapamil
B. Thyroid surgery
C. Hyperventilation
D. Malabsorption

Ans: (A)

Ca +ve channel blocker does not cause *Tetany.*

Tetany:

- Low ionized calcium concentrations cause increased excitability of peripheral nerves.
- Latent Tetany may be present when sign of rest tetany are lacking. It is best recognized by eliciting **Trousseau's sign.**
- A less specific sign of hypocalcaemia is that described by **Chvostek** in which tapping on the branches of the facial nerve as they emerge from the parotid gland produces twitching of the facial muscles.

(Reference: 19th Edition, Davidson's Page No. 717)

Q.10. Which of the following is not a usual feature of right middle cerebral artery territory infarct?

A. Aphasia
B. Hemiparesis
C. Facial weakness
D. Dysarthria

Ans: (A)

Aphasia is a manifestation of dominant parietal lobe involvement. Dominant hemisphere in right handed persons is left hemisphere and thus a right middle cerebral artery infarct indicates non dominant parietal lobe involvement. Aphasia will not be a manifestation because an infarction in middle cerebral artery distribution on the right side will affect the non dominant parietal lobe. (Left parietal lobe).

Clinical manifestation of the middle cerebral Artery involvement:

- *Contralateral hemiplegia*: Motor cortex involvement
- *Contralateral hemianaesthesia*: Sensory cortex Involvement
- *Homonymous hemianopia:* Optic radiation Involvement

(Reference: Harrison 16th Edition. Page No. 2381)

MEDICINE

Q.11. All are causes of flapping tremor *except*:

A. Hepatic encephalopathy
B. Uremic encephalopathy
C. Carbondioxide narcosis
D. Thyrotoxicosis

Ans: (D)

ASTEREXIS: Is the flapping tremor seen in metabolic disturbances is as the result of intermittent failure of the parietal mechanism which maintains posture. There is sudden periods of cessation of muscle contraction best seen when the patient arms are extended in front.

Causes of Asterexis

- Renal/liver failure
- Hypercapnia
- Drug toxicity
- Acute focal parietal or thalamic lesions.

Q.12. A 40-year-old male develops excessive hyperventilation ABG reveals PH-7.5 Pco2 -24 mmHg Po2-88mmHg. Diagnosis is:

A. Respiratory Alkalosis
B. Metabolic Alkalosis
C. Respiratory acidosis
D. Metabolic acidosis

Ans: (A)

There is Alkalosis (PH - 7.5) and Co2 is low (Alkalosis) change in Co2 with change in PH and thus the primary cause is Respiratory. The acid base disturbance is thus primary respiratory Alkalosis.

Q.13. True about pancoast Tumor all *except*:

A. Lower lobe carcinoma
B. Squamous cell carcinoma
C. Causes Horner syndrome
D. Located in the Apex

Ans: (A)

- Pan-coast tumor occurs in Association with Lung cancer (Epidermoid or squamous cell carcinoma)
- The tumor is usually located in the apex of lung, grows locally to involve the brachial plexus. Usually there is involvement of 8th cervical, 1st and 2nd thoracic nerves. This causes shoulder pain that radiates in the ulnar distribution of the arm.
- It also causes Horner's syndrome:
  - Unilateral ptosis
  - Miosis
  - *Ispilateral Anhydrosis*

Remember

- Most common variety of Lung ca in India—*Squamous cell carcinoma*
- Most common variety in world—*Adeno carcinoma*
- Histological variety that cavitates—*Squamous cell carcinoma*
- Most common site for metastasis from ca lung- liver, Variety most responsive to chemotherapy —*Small cell carcinoma*
- Variety with best prognosis—*Squamous cell carcinoma*

MEDICINE

Most common variety with cushing syndrome—*Small cell carcinoma*

Most common endocrinal gland to be involved by metastasis —*Adrenal carcinoma*

Ca which metastasize to opposite lung—*Adeno carcinoma*

Most common endocrinal gland to be involved by metastasis —*Adrenal gland*

Remember:

Most common secondaries metastasize to Lymph node and after that is liver.

Q.14. Most common CNS manifestation of HIV Infection is:

A. Acute Meningitis

B. Encephalopathy

C. Vacuolar myelopathy

D. Dementia

Ans: (D)

- HIV Encephalopathy also called HIV - Associated dementia or AIDS dementia.
- This is generally a late complication of HIV infection, it can be seen patients with CD4 count >350 cells.
- HIV encephalopathy is a *sub-cortical dementia* while
- Alzheimer's is a cortical dementia
- Alzheimer's disease is the most common cause of dementia in elderly.
- Most important risk factor for Alzheimer's disease is age.

(Reference: P. No. 1116, Harrison-16th Edition)

Q.15. All are the risk factors for coronary artery disease *except*:

A. LDL **B.** HDL

C. Smoking **D.** Hypertension

Ans: (B)

Some important risk factors for Atherosclerosis:

Fixed

- Family history

MEDICINE

- Age
- Sex (male)

Modifiable

- Smoking
- Haemostatic variables
- Hypertension
- Sedentary life styles
- Lipid disorders
- Obesity
- D.M
- Diet

Atherosclerotic vascular disease may manifest as coronary heart disease, cerebrovascular disease or peripheral vascular disease. Occult coronary artery disease is common in those who present with other forms of atherosclerotic vascular disease. So risk factors for atherosclerosis is also are the risk factors for CAD.

(Reference: Page No. 442, Davidson-19th edition)

Q.16. Lung carcinoma most common associated with:

A. Asbestosis
B. Silicosis
C. Byssinosis
D. Beryllium

Ans: (A)

Remember some important points.

- *Silicosis*—currently the most prevalent chronic occupational disease in the world
- Silicosis is associated with an increased susceptibility to Tuberculosis. The radiological feature—*EGG SHELL calcification in the hilar lymphnodes.*
- *Berylliosis* cause an interstitial granulomatous disease similar to Sarcoidosis.
- The most dangerous particles to cause Pneumoconiosis from 1 to 5 micrometer in diameter because they may reach in the

terminal small airways, air sacs and settle in their lining.

- Cotton dust is associated with *Byssinosis.*
- Sugarcane dust is associated with *Bagassois*

(Reference: Page No. 733, Robinson-7th edition)

Q.17. MCTD includes all the following *except*:

A. Polymyositis **B.** RA
C. Osteoarthritis **D.** Systemic sclerosis

Ans: (C)

Mixed connective tissue diseases (MCTD) are sometimes used to describe the disease seen in a group of patient who are identified clinically by the coexistence of features suggestive of SLE. Polymyositis, Rheumatoid arthritis and systemic sclerosis and serologically by high titres of antibodies to RNP Particle containing UI RNP.

Two factors are important in lending distinctiveness to MCTD are:

- The paucity of renal disease.
- Extremely good response to corticosteroid.

Some important points about connective tissue disorder:

- Antinuclear antibodies in autoimmune disease.
- Anti double stranded DNA→*SLE (more specific than anti SM antibody).*
- Anti Histone Antibodies→*Drug induced lupus erythrocytosis*
- Anti **sm** antibody→*SLE*
- Anti DNA topoisomerase antibody→*Systemic sclerosis*
- Antibodies of Ribonucleoprotein Antigen containing ULRNP→*Mixed connective tissue disorder.*
- Antimitochondrial antibody→*Primary biliary cirrhosis.*

Q.18. Microangiopathic Hemolytic anemia seen in:

A. HUS
B. HTN

C. SLE
D. All

Ans: (D)

Micro-angiopathic Hemolytic anemia occurs when red blood cells are forced to squeeze through abnormally narrowed small vessels. Narrowing is most often caused by fibrin deposition in association with DIC.

Other causes of micro-angiopathic hemolytic anemia are:

- Malignant hypertension
- SLE
- Thrombotic Thrombocytopenic purpura.
- HUS
- Disseminated cancer.

The common feature among all these disorders is a Micro vascular Lesion that cause mechanical injury to circulating Red blood cells.

In blood smear in the form of red cell fragments (schisocytes) burr cells, helmet cells and triangle cells are seen.

Some important Point:

- Most common cause of Anemia in world is Iron deficient Anemia.
- Most sensitive and specific test for diagnosis of from deficiency is serum ferritin levels.
- Hyper segmented neutrophilis are a feature of megaloblastic anemia and not iron deficient anemia.

Cause of microcytic hypochromic anemia
Mnemonics: Tiny CLIPS

- Iron deficient Anemia
- Thalassaemia
- Sideroblastic anemia,
- Lead poisoning
- Anemia of chronic disease.
- Pyridoxin deficit anemia.

Q.19. "a" wave in JVP indicates:

A. Atrial systole
B. Ventricular systole

C. Atrial relaxation
D. Tricuspid regurgitation

Ans: (A)

A wave: Are positive waves due to distention produced by right atrial contraction

Large a waves: Indicate atrium is contracting against increased resistance tricuspid stenosis, pulmonary stenosis, pulmonary hypertension.

Cannon S waves

Regularly: During junctional rhythm. *Irregularly:* complete Heart Block.

Absent a waves: Atrial Fibrillation

Q.20. Anti mitochondrial Ab seen typically in:

A. Primary Biliary cirrhosis
B. Hepatitis B
C. Hepatitis C
D. Hepatitis A

Ans: (A)

Primary Biliary cirrhosis is a disease characterized by chronic inflammation and fibrous obliteration of intrahepatic bile ductioles due to an unknown (primary) stimulus.

Etiology

PBC is believed to due to an autoimmune etiology as it is often associated with other auto immune disorders such as

- CREST syndrome: Calcinosis, Raynaud's phenomena, Esophageal dysmotility, Sclerodactily, Telangiectasia
- Sicca syndrome
- Autoimmune thyroiditis
- Renal tubular acidosis

Anti mitochondrial antibody (IgG is positive)

Clinical feature

- Most patients are asymptomatic.
- Pruritis is commonest/earliest symptom
- Jaundice

Deficiency of fat soluble vitamin due to malabsorption leads to:

Vit D deficiency→ Bone pain—Osteomyelitis

Vit K deficiency→bleeding bruising
Vit A deficiency→Night Blindness
Xanthelisma and Xanthomas are due to elevation of serum lipids.

Lab finding

Increased Serum alkaline phosphates.
Positive mitochondrial antibody sensitive and specific.

Q.21. Hepatorenal syndrome characterised by all *except*:

A. No proteinuria
B. Normal intrinsic kidney.
C. Liver failure
D. Urine osmolality less than plasma osmolality

Ans: (D)

Renal failure consequent on liver failure can occur in cirrhosis. The kidney's they are intrinsically normal and renal failure is thought to result from altered systemic blood flow including diminished renal blood flow:

- It occurs in advanced cirrhosis at most always and ascites
- Absence of proteinuria or abnormal urinary sediment.
- Urine sodium excretion below 10mmol/day.
- Serum Na+ concentration < 130 m Eq/l.
- Urinary osmolality greater than plasma osmolality.
- Urine volume < 500 ml/day.

Q.22. In infant LRTI is MC caused by:

A. Streptococci
B. RSV Viruses
C. H. Influenza
D. Mycoplasma

Ans: (B)

RSV virus is m/c cause of bronchiolitis in Infants. Doc- **Ribavirin**. Epiglottis is most commonly caused by H. Influenzae.

Some Important points:

Encephalitis→it is the Inflammation of the brain parenchyma

Meningitis→is an acute purulent infection with in the subarachnoid space.The meninges, the subarachnoid space and brain parenchyma are all frequently involved in the inflammatory reaction with meningo-encephalitis.

- The most common cause of sporadic viral encephalitis →**HSV -I**
- The most common cause of Epidemic viral encephalitis→**Arborirus**
- Japanese encephalitis virus is an arbovirus is one of the most common causes of encephalitis outbreak.
- The most common cause of viral meningitis is→**Enterovirus**

Q.23. Megaloblastic anemia is caused by:

A. Diphyllobothrium latum

B. H-NaNa

C. Taenia saginata

D. Echinococcus granulosis.

Ans: (A)

Habitat: Adult worm lives in small intestine (ileum or jejunum) of man D.Latum is the longest tapeworm found in man.

Life cycle:

The worm passes its life cycle in one definitive host and Two intermediate host.

Definitive host: Man is the main definitive host

Intermediate host:

First intermediate host: Small copepods mainly of genra Diaptomus and Cyclops

Second intermediate host: Freshwater Fishes.

Humans become infected when they eat undercooked raw or lightly salted meat or roe from infected freshwater fishes.

Pathogenicity:

Most human infections are caused by only one tape worm and cause no or very vague ill effects.

MEDICINE

Patient may develop fatigue, weakness, diarrhoea and numbness of extremities. Some Patient develops mechanical obstruction. In few cases pernicious anemia may develop due to B12 deficiency. D. Latum has been shown to absorb as much as 80-100% of a single oral dose of vit-B12 thereby competing with the host for this important vitamin.

Treatment of choice:

Niclosamide and praziquantel

Important:

Vit B_{12} Absorb in the **ILEUM.**

Iron is absorbed in the **Duodenum.**

Q.24. Nephrocalcinosis is a feature of:

A. Primary Hyperparathyroidism

B. Medullary cystic kidney

C. Vitamin C Intoxication

D. Pseudohypoparathyroidism

Ans: (A)

Most Important Point:

- Patient with Hyperparathyroidism are asymptomatic.
- Manifestation of Hyperparathyroidism involve primarily the kidney and skeletal system.
- Kidney involvement due to deposition of calcium in renal parenchyma or to recurrent Nephrolithiasis.
- Renal stones are usually composed of either calcium oxalate with calcium phosphate.
- Nephrocalcinosis may also cause decreased renal function and phosphate retention.

Another Important Question

Q.25. Asymptomatic hypercalcemia in 30-year-old young male is due to:

A. Occult Primary Malignancy

B. Primary Hyperparathyroidism

C. Familial Hypocalciuria

D. Hypernephroma

Ans: (B)

The most common presentation in a patient with Primary hyperparathyroidism is asymptomatic hypercalcamia.

Q.26. Carotid Massage is useful in:

A. Ventricular extrasystole

B. Atrial flutter

C. PSVT

D. Ventricular fibrillation

Ans: (C)

Other Important Point:

- The most effective T/T of atrial flutter is D.C. cardioversion.
- Drug of choice in PSVT with adenosine.
- Agent of second choice in PSVT is Beta Blockers.
- Carotid massage is useful in **PSVT and AV Nodal Recurrent tachycardia.**

Q.27. Zinc deficiency is seen in all *except*:

A. Inflammatory bowel disease

B. Malabsorption syndrome

C. Sickle cell anemia

D. T.B.

Ans: (D)

Mild zinc deficiency has been described in many diseases including diabetes mellitus. AIDS, Cirrhosis, Alcoholism, Inflammatory bowel, Disease malabsorption syndrome and sickle cell anemia.

T.B. is not mentioned in Harrison.

(Reference: Harrison 16th Edition, Page No. 409)

Q.28. Most common cause of Hypovolaemic shock is:

A. Haemorrhage

B. Gram -ve Bacteria

C. Tension Pneumothorax

D. Gram +ve

Ans: (A)

Hypovolumic shock:

This is most common form of shock results either from the loss of red blood cells more and plasma from hemorrhage.

Classification of Shock

a. Hypovolumic shock
   - Loss of blood—Hemorrhagic shock
   - Loss of plasma as in burns shock
   - Loss of fluid—dehydration as in gastroenteritis.

b. Septic shock
   - M/c common due to gram -ve organism.

c. Cardiogenic shock
   - Due to pump failure as in myocardial infection, pericardial effusion, pulmonary embolism.

d. Neurogenic shock

e. Anaphylactic shock

M/c due to penicillin drugs, toxin etc

Q.29. Not a cause of Cor Pulmonale:

A. Mitral stenosis

B. Intermittent pulmonary embolism

C. COPD

D. Kyphoscoliosis.

Ans: (B)

- Recurrent pulmonary thromboembolism is the cause of cor pulmonale. Cor pulmonale is frequently called as pulmonary Hypertensive Heart disease consists of right ventricular hypertrophy.
- Cor pulmonale may be acute or chronic
- Acute cor pulmonale can follow massive pulmonary embolism.
- Chronic cor pulmonale usually implies right ventricular hypertrophy and dilation secondary to prolonged pressure overload caused by obstruction of pulmonary arteries and arterioles.

- There is long list of disorders predisposing for cor pulmonale. But remember some important conditions.

Disease of the pulmonary parenchyma.

- COPD
- Cystic fibrosis
- Bronchiectasis

Disorders of the pulmonary vessels.

- Recurrent pulmonary thromboembolism
- Primary pulmonary hypertension.
- Extensive pulmonary arteritis eg .
- (wegener's granulomatosis)
- **Drug:** Toxin or radiation Induced
- Vascular obstruction

Disorders affecting chest movement

- Kyphoscoliosis
- Marked obesity (pick wickian syndrome)
- Neuromuscular disease.

Q.30. Pretibial myxoedema is seen in:

A. Thyrotoxicosis
B. Myxoedema
C. Follicular ca
D. Papillary ca thyroid

Ans: (A)

Grave's disease consist of triad

1. Diffuse thyroid enlargement
2. Opthalmopathy
3. Pretibial myxoedema

Thyrotoxicosis is a feature of graves disease.

Pretibial myxoedema is a misnomer. It is not seen in myxoedema.

Antithyroid of choice in pregnancy is propylthiouracil.

Q.31. Exudative pleural effusion seen in all *except:*

A. Acute Pancreatitis
B. SLE
C. CCF
D. Tuberculosis

Ans: (C)

Transudative effusion: Pleural fluid accumulates is a result of increased hydrostatic pressure or decreased osmotic pressure. Eg: Cardiac, liver and renal failure.

Exudative effusion: Due to increased microvascular permeability due to disease of the pleural surface itself or injury.

Eg: Tuberculosis, malignant disease, pulmonary infarction, Rheumatoid Disease, SLE, Acute Pancreatitis.

(Reference: Davidson's 19th Edition, Page No. 502)

Q.32. Nephrocalcinosis is seen in all *except*:

A. Hyperparathyroidism
B. Multiple myeloma
C. Malignancy
D. Rickets

Ans: (D)

Almost all the Hypercalcemic conditions leads to nephrocalcinosis.

The Hypercalcemic conditions are:

- Hyperparathyroidism
- Multiple myeloma.
- Vitamin D intoxication
- Metastatic bone diseases.
- Milk alkali syndrome.
- Malignancy (eg. Lung, Breast, renal)
- Thyrotoxicosis

So the vitamin deficiency (Rickets) doesn't leads to hypercalcemia, only vitamin D intoxication causes hypercalcemia.

(Reference: Davidson 19th Edition, P. No. 516)

Q.33. Hypotonia not seen in:

A. Hypokalemia
B. Deep sleep
C. LMNL
D. Parkinsonism

Ans: (D)

Hypotonia is also known as Flaccidity.

Hypotonia is usually associated with Hyporeflexia, Muscle weakness and wasting.

Cause of hypotonia:

- LMN Lesion.
- Posterior column lesion (Tabes dorsalis)
- Myopathy
- Down's syndrome
- Rickets
- Deep sleep
- Hypokalemia or hyperkalaemia

Hypertonia is of two types:

Plasticity (pyramidal lesion)

Rigidity (extra pyramidal lesion)

Hypertonia is seen in:

- UMN lesion (Claspknife spasticity)
- Extrapyramidal lesion except chorea (lead pipe or cogwheel rigidity) eg: Parkinsonism.
- Tetanus
- Strychnine poisoning
- Tetany
- Decerebrate rigidity.

(Reference: Kundu 4th edition, page no: 160)

MEDICINE

Q.34. A sewer worker admitted with fever, Jaundice and Renal failure the most appropriate diagnosis will be:

A. HVS

B. Leprosporosis

C. Renal failure

D. Legionella

Ans: (B)

The patient in this question is a case of Weil's syndrome or Leptospirosis or Ictar haemorrhagicus fever.

Clue to diagnosis are:

a. Sewer worker

b. Jaundice

Sewer worker: Leptosporosis is transmitted to human being through water contaminated with urine of carrier animals. Leptospirae from this water enters the body through cuts or abrasions on skin or through intact mucosa of Mouth, Nose or Conjunctiva.

Characteristic features of weil's syndrome are:
- Fever
- Jaundice
- Renal failure

Serological test: MAT (Microscopic agglutination Test) is used for diagnosis.

Q.35. In Crohn's disease not seen:

A. Stricture
B. Fistula
C. Skip lesion
D. Pseudopolyp

Ans: (D)

Clonic involvement with ulcerative colitis is characterized by extensive broad based ulceration of the mucosa in the distal colon and through its length. Pseudopolyps are created by bulging upwards of isolated islands of regenerating mucosa. Pseudopolyps are a feature of ulcerative colitis.

Features	*Crohn's disease*	*Ulcerative colitis*
1. Distribution	Segmental with skip areas	Continuous without skip area
2. Location	Commonly terminal ileum	Commonly Rectum, Sigmoid colon
3. Pseudopolyps	Rarely seen	Commonly present
4. Extent	Usually involves the entire thickness of allocated segment of bowel wall	Superficial mucosal ulcer without fissure
Complication:		
1. Fistula formation	Internal and external fistula in 10% cases	Externally rare
2. Fibrous stricture	Common	Never
3. Toxic megacolon	Absent	Present
4. Named Feature	Cobble stone appearance	Pseudopolyps

Q.36. Differential diagnosis of chylous ascites are all *except:*

A. Tuberculosis
B. Hypothyroidism
C. Filariasis
D. Lymphoma

Ans: (B)

1. *Chylous*—Turbid creamy or milky peritoneal fluid due to presence of lymph. It shows sudden standing fat globules and contain a large amount of triglyceride. **Ether** dissolves the turbidity of chylous ascites.
2. *Chyliform ascites*—Turbid due to large number of Leucocyte, Degenerated cells or Tumor cells. Addition of alkali clears the turbidity.
3. *Pseudochylous Ascites*—Turbid fluid due to increased amount of Lecthin, Globulin and Calcium phosphate in the ascitic fluid.

Causes of Chylous ascites:

- Tuberculosis
- Filariasis
- Trauma to the abdomen
- Intra abdominal malignancy
- Nephrotic syndrome
- Congenital abnormality in the lymphatics or obstruction to the thoracic duct.

These are the differential diagnosis of the chylous ascites.

Q.37. Exudate are seen in all *except*:

A. CHF
B. TB
C. Malignancy
D. Uremia

Ans: (A)

How to differentiate transudate from exudates:

	Transudate	*Exudate*
1. Appearance	Clear does not clot on standing or purulent often	Turbid straw colour haemorrhagic, chylous, Mucionous clots on standing.
2. Specific gravity	<1.016	>1.016
3. Proteins	<2.5g/dl	>2.5g/dl
4. Cells	Endothelial cells or Mesothelial cells and occasionally lymphocytes are seen.	Lymphocyte, Neutrophils or malignant cells

Causes of Transudate and Exudate ascites:

Transudate	*Exudate*
1. Cirrhosis of liver	1. Peritonitis * Pyogenic * TB * Malignant * Spontaneous bacterial peritonitis
2. CCF	2. Pancreatic ascites
3. Nephrotic syndrome	3. Lymphoma or leukemia
4. Pericardial effusion	4. Injury or obstruction to thoracic duct.
5. Myxoedema	
6. Constrictive pericarditis	

Q.38. Pregnant lady presents with fulminate hepatitis, most common cause is:

A. Hepatitis A

B. Hepatitis B

C. Hepatitis C

D. Hepatitis D

Ans: (B)

- The most feared complication of viral hepatitis is fulminate hepatitis (Massive hepatic necrosis).
- Fulminate hepatitis is primarily seen in hepatitis B and D; As well as in hepatitis E.

MEDICINE

- Rare fulminate cases of hepatitis A occur primarily in **older adults** in person with chronic liver disease.
- Fulminate hepatitis is seen rarely in hepatitis C.
- Hepatitis E can be complicated by fetal fulminate hepatitis in 1-2% of all cases and in up to 20% of cases occurring in pregnant women.
- Hepatitis B accounts for >50% of fulminate hepatitis cases.
- Patients with simultaneous acute hepatitis B and D do not necessarily experience higher mortality rate than do patients with acute hepatitis B alone.

From above points what I concluded:

- Fulminate hepatitis - Because of Hepatitis A, is primarily in **older and adult** patients. So from the choice it excluded.
- Fulminate hepatitis is rarely seen in Hepatitis C but it is the most common cause of chronic viral Hepatitis. So this is also excluded from the choice.
- Fulminate hepatitis because of Hepatitis E is strongly associated with pregnant lady but in question Hepatitis E is not in choice.
- Hepatitis B accounts for more than 50% is of Fulminate hepatitis.
- Patients with simultaneous acute hepatitis B and D do not necessarily experience higher mortality rate than do patients with acute hepatitis B alone, so Hepatitis D also excluded.

After going through number of books my answer will favor to Hepatitis B.

(Reference: Harrison 16th Edition, Page No. 1834)

MEDICINE

FIFTEEN

Ophthalmology

Q.1. Interstitial Keratitis most commonly cause by:

A. Streptococcus infection
B. Sarcoidosis
C. Syphilis
D. Kerato conjunctivitis sicca

Ans: (C)

Interstitial Keratitis - Inflammation of corneal stroma **without** primary involvement of **epithelium** or **endothelium.**

Most commonly associated with congenital syphilis (90%) than acquired syphilis.

Sarcoidosis also causes the *interstitial keratitis*.

Keratoconjunctivitis sicca is the cause of Filamentary *Keratitis*.

Q.2. Scleritis is most commonly associated with:

A. Rheumatoid Arthritis
B. Tuberculosis
C. Staphylococcal infection
D. Thyrotoxicosis

Ans: (A)

All the given choice is associated with scleritis, but most commonly associated with **Rheumatoid arthritis.**

Scleritis is also associated with Wegener's granulomatosis, SLE, ankylosing spondylitis, syphilis, sarcoidosis and Leprosy.

Q.3. Acute Anterior uveitis is associated with HLA:

A. HLA - A 28 **B.** HLA B27
C. HLA DR3 **D.** HLA A3

Ans: (B)

Try to remember about **HLA B27**

1. Ankylosing spondylitis
2. Juvenile rheumatoid Arthritis
3. Psoriatic Arthritis
4. Reactive Arthritis
5. Acute Anterior Uveitis
6. Reiter's syndrome

HLA A3 → *Haemochromatosis*

HLA DR4, DR3 → *Type I diabetes mellitus*

HLA - B8 → *Myasthenia gravis*

HLA B5 → *Polycystic Kidney, Ulcerative colitis, Bechet's diseases*

Q.4. 1 mm increase in axial length leads to Increase the Power by:

A. 1D **B.** 2 D

C. 3 D **D.** 4 D

Ans: (C)

Q.5. Light Reflex is carried through:

A. Ciliary nerve **B.** V C.N

C. VII C.N **D.** Optic nerve

Ans: (D)

(Reference: Textbook of Clinical Neuroanatomy Vishram Singh Page No. 289)

Light Reflex or Pupillary reflex.

Pathway of reflex.

- *Afferent Limb:* The visual impulses travel through the optic nerve, optic chiasma & optic tract to terminate in the pretectal nucleus. Then impulses from pretectal nucleus pass to the parasympathetic nuclei (Edinger westphal nuclei) of third cranial nerve.
- *Efferent Limb*: The impulses from the Edinger westphal nucleus pass bilaterally along the occulomotor nerve to the ciliary ganglion. The postganglionic parasympathetic fibres travel along the short ciliary nerve to supply the sphincter pupillae muscles of the iris leading to constriction of pupils of both the eyes.

Light stimulus→Optic nerve→Optic tract →Pretectal nucleus →
Sphincter pupillae←Ciliary ganglion←Occulomotor nerve← Edinger westphal nucleus ↲
↑
Short ciliary nerve

Q.6. Most common cause of vision loss in HIV:

A. CMV retinitis

B. Toxoplasma

C. Herpes simplex

D. Candida

Ans: (A)

CMV causes opportunistic infection of eye in Immuno-compromised patients. One of the **most devastating** consequences of HIV infection is **CMV retinitis.**

Ocular lesions of AIDS:

- *Retinal micro-vasculopathy, which gives multiple* ***cotton wool spots****.*
- *Usual ocular infection are mostly by herpes zoster opthalmicus, Herpes simplex and Toxoplasmosis.*
- *Opportunistic Infection of eye is mostly in HIV or leukemia, by CMV.*
- *Unusual neoplasma that is kaposi sarcoma and Burkit's Lymphoma.*

(Reference: Page No. 417, A.K. Khurana Page No. 1119, Harrison 16th Edition)

Q.7. Dendritic ulcer seen in:

A. Candida

B. Trauma

C. Herpes Simplex

D. CMV

Ans: (C)

Dendritic ulcer is a typical lesion of recurrent epithelial keratitis. The ulcer is irregular, zig-zag linear branching shape.

Q.8. Axial length of the eye ball is _____ mm:

A. 24 mm **B.** 23.5 mm

C. 75 mm **D.** 23 mm

Ans: (A)

- Dimension's of An Adult Eyeball. Axial length (A-P diameter) = **24 mm.**
- Horizontal diameter = **23.5 mm**
- Vertical diameter = **23 mm**
- Circumference = **75 mm**
- Volume = **6.5 ml**
- Weight = **7 gm.**

Q.9. Rosette shaped cataract seen in:

A. Trauma
B. Wilson's disease
C. Galactosemia
D. Diabetic patient

Ans: (a)

Types of cataract seen in different disease:

- Wilson's disease →***Sunflower cataract***
- Diabetes→***Snow Flake appearance cataract***
- Trauma→***Rosette cataract***
- Galactosemia→***Oil drop cataract***
- Rubella →***Salt & Pepper appearance***
- In Myotonica dystrophica →***Posterior Subcapsular stellate opacities in lens (Christmas tree pattern)***
- In Tetany→***Crystaline flakes opacities***

Q.10. Muscle most commonly involved in Thyroid Opthalmopathy is:

A. Medial Rectus
B. Lateral Rectus
C. Superior Rectus
D. Inferior Rectus

Ans: (D)

In Grave's disease, Restrictive thyroid myopathy - IR most commonly involved.

Other clinical features of grave's disease:

➢ *Eyelid Retraction*
- Lid Retraction - Dalrymple's sign
- Upper lid lag on down gaze – Vongrafer sign
- Staring and Frightened appearance of eye - Kocher's sign
- Poor convergence - Mobius sign

OPHTHALMOLOGY

➢ *Infiltrative Opthalmopathy*

– Enlargement of EOM 8 times than normal size.

→ Restrictive myopathy

➢ *Proptosis - U/L or B/L*

➢ *Dysthyroid optic Neuropathy*

- Due to compression of Optic nerve
- Central / Paracentral scotoma
- Impaired colour vision.

Q.11. Superior Oblique muscle is supplied by:

A. V C.N

B. VI C.N

C. III C.N

D. IV C.N

Ans: (D)

There are six Extraocular muscles, they are

1. Medial rectus—III C.N
2. Lateral rectus—VI C.N
3. Superior rectus—III C.N
4. Inferior rectus—III C.N
5. Superior Oblique—IV C.N
6. Inferior Oblique—III C.N

All muscle is supplied by III C.N, Except LR which is by VI C.N and SO which is by IV C.N.

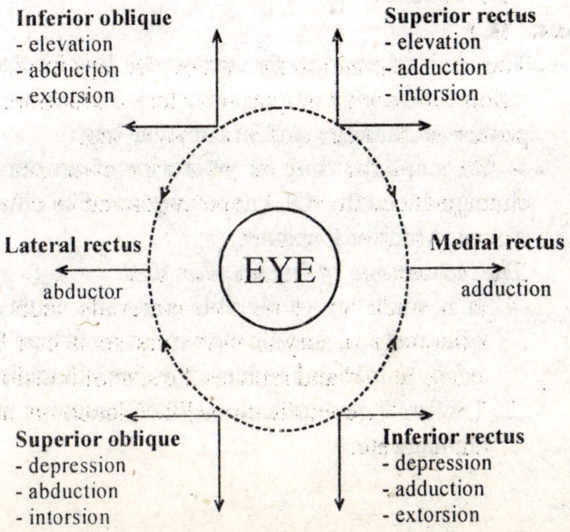

Q.12. Maximum No. of cones are seen in:

A. Fovea centralis
B. Blind spot
C. Macula Lutea
D. Optic disc

Ans: (A)

Fovea centralis: In this area no rods, cones are tightly packed. All other retinal layers are absent in this region. In foveal region surrounding the foveal the axons of the cones are arranged obliquely to reach the margin of the fovea K/as **Henle's layer.**

Optic disc:

All retinal layers end here except nerve fibers which runs into optic nerve.

Macula:

Yellow spot situated at the posterior pole temporal to optic disc.

(Reference: Page No. 250, Khurana 3rd Edition)

Q.13. Ideal site for the intra-ocular lens is:

A. Iris Clip
B. Anterior Chamber
C. Posterior Chamber
D. Vitreous

Ans: (C)

- The optimal position for intraocular lens implantation following extra capsular lens extraction, is posterior chamber and in capsular bag.
- If the capsular bag or posterior chamber is damaged then the IOL can be implanted in ciliary sulcus Anterior Capsules.

The Advantage of Intraocular lens:

1. It is made up of flexible materials such as silicone and acrylic polymers so it can be easily folded and reduces the size of incision.
2. Lowers the complications like Glaucoma, iris damage etc.

Q.14. Most serious complication after traumatic injury to one eye

A. Optic Neuritis

B. Sympathetic Opthalmitis

C. Glaucoma

D. Endopthalmitis

Ans: (B)

- It is a B/L granulomatous uveitis, following penetrating injuries.
- Develops within 3 wks to 12 wks after injury to eye.
- First **Symptom** is **photophobia**
- First **sign** is **retrolental Flare**
- **Dalen—Fuchs's nodules** are soft yellow white exudates seen in deep layer.

Q.15. Laser used for posterior capsulotomy after cataract iridotomy vitreolysis.

A. Argon green

B. ND - YAG

C. Diode Laser

D. Excimer

Ans: (B)

These are the types of laser used in ophthalmology.

- ND YAG→*Posterior capsulotomy in after cataract iridotomy vitreolysis.*
- Nd YAG (frequency double)→*Retinal photocoagulation, cyclo-photocoagulation.*
- Argon Green→*Trabeculoplasty, iridoplasty, pupillomydriasis, Retinal Photocoagulation.*
- Diode Laser and krypton Red→*Retinal photocoagulation*
- Excimer (Argon fluoride)→*LASIK, LASEK, Keratometry.*

Remember:

Retinal photocoagulation mainly used diabetic Retinopathy, Argon green lasers are most widely used.

Q.16. Treatment of choice in Angle closure Glaucoma:

A. Pilocarpine **B.** Surgical iridotomy
C. Laser iridotomy **D.** Trabeculectomy

Ans: (C)

Treatment Plan: includes initial medical therapy followed by surgery.

Medical therapy

1. First—Acetazolamide 1/v is given followed by oral therapy.
2. Topical pilocarpine is used only after high IOP is brought down to under 40mmHg.

Surgical therapy

Nd YAG laser peripheral iridotomy, once IOP is under control, peripheral iridotomy is done for both eyes.
Trabeculectomy is done in case of failure of peripheral iridotomy.

Q.17. Dendritic ulcer seen in:

A. Herpes zoster
B. Adeno Virus
C. Chlamydia Trachoma
D. Herpes simplex

Ans: (D)

Dendritic ulcer is the pathognomic feature of Herpes simplex keratitis.
The other ocular manifestation Herpes Simplex

- Blepharitis
- Conjunctivitis
- Iridocyclitis
- Keratitis

Treatment: Topical antiviral and antibiotics to prevent secondary bacterial infections.

Adenovirus

→ cause **swimming pool conjunctivitis.**
Chlamydia trachoma causes **keratoconjunctivitis.**

(Reference: Page No. 124, Khurana- 3rd Edition)

Q.18. Tractional Retinal detachment is seen in:

A. Vitreous loss after surgery
B. Diabetes mellitus
C. Renal Hypertension
D. Ocular diseases

Ans: (B)

Retinal detachment→separation of Neurosensory Retina proper from the pigment epithelium.

Classified into 3 types:

1. Rhegmatogenous—Primary Retinal detachment
2. Tractional retinal detachment
3. Exudative Retinal detachment—secondary detachment

The cause of Tractional retinal detachment → post traumatic retraction, proliferate diabetic retinopathy, Post hemorrhagic retinitis.

Renal Hypertension and ocular disease are the cause of Exudative detachment.

Q.19. In Direct Opthalmoscopy image is magnified:

A. 5 times　　**B.** 10 times
C. 15 times　　**D.** 20 times

Ans: (C)

Indirect opthalmoscopy magnification of **5 times, direct of 15 times.**

(Reference: Page No. 35, Khurana)

Q.20. Leukocoria is the feature of:

A. Retinoblastoma　　**B.** Glaucoma
C. Cataract　　**D.** Trachoma

Ans: (A)

1. Leuckocoria also called as **yellowish - white pupillary reflex** or **Amaurotic cat's eye appearance.**
2. It is the most common resenting feature of **Retinoblastoma.**
3. Retinoblastoma **most common tumor of eye.**
4. **Strabismus is the second most common feature.**

SIXTEEN

Surgery

Q.1. Painful tender and non reducible sac through inguinal canal with absent cough reflex you seen in:

A. Obstructed hernia

B. Strangulated hernia

C. Ricter's hernia

D. Incarcerated hernia

Ans: (B)

Stangulated hernia:

Irreducibility, obstruction and arrest of blood supply to the contents.

Accompanied with pain and vomiting, obviously there is no cough impulse.

Obstructed hernia:

Irreducibility and intestinal obstruction, obstruction due to occlusion of lumen of the bowel.

Incarcerated hernia:

Often used as an alternative to obstructed hernia, but to the precise if indicates that a portion of colon is the content of sac and is blocked with feaces.

Ricter's hernia:

The content of sac is a portion of the circumference of the intestine.

Littre's hernia:

When the content is mickel's diverticulum.

(Reference: Page No. 1091, S. Das 3rd Edition)

Q.2. Most common mode of spread of Gall bladder carcinoma:

A. Transcoelemic spread.

B. Lymphogenic spread

C. Haematogenic spread

D. Direct spread.

Ans: (D)

Gall bladder carcinoma: The main route of spread are:

- Direct infiltration
- Lymphatic spread
- Vascular spread
- Intraductal spread

Direct infiltration is the **most common first mode of involvement**, second through lymphaticus.

Most common type of Gallbladder carcinoma —*Serous adenocarcinoma.*

Most common site - *Fundus of Gallbladder.*

(Reference: Page No. 1920, S. Das 3rd Edition)

Q.3. Thimble bladder is seen in:

A. Acute tuberculosis

B. Chronic tuberculosis

C. Neurogenic bladder

D. Schistosomiasis

Ans: (B)

When the tuberculosis involves the urinary bladder, it results in FIBROSIS. So, it become small contracted, ineffectively functioning. Storage capacity is lost resulting in intractable frequency with few drops of urine.

There is bleeding and painful micturition which called STRANGURY. There is also severe pain in supra pubic region which referred to tip of penis. Such a bladder is called **thimble bladder**. Treatment of **thimble bladder** is **ileocysto-plasty**.

Remember

Golf hole ureter is seen in **Tuberculosis of bladder**.

Putty kidney → caseous material present in kidney because of Tuberculosis of parenchyma kidney.

Cement kidney → when calcification of putty kidney takes place, it is known as cement kidney; which on X-ray appears as calculi (Pseudo calculi).

Scistosomiasia of the bladder:

- S.Haematobium - affecting mainly the bladder.
- S.Japanicum - affecting mainly the liver and small intestine.
- S.Mansoni - affecting mainly the large intestine.
- S.Haematobium infection leads to granulamatous heamaturia and later granulomas calcify and develop a **sandy** appearance.
- If calcification is severe and it takes place through out the bladder wall, On X-ray film it appears as **fetal head** in pelvis.
- Scistosomiasis also leads to contraction the bladder.
- It is a risk factor for bladder carcinoma. It is a **squamous cell** carcinoma but **not the Transitional cell carcinoma.**

(Reference: Page No. 547, K.Rajgopal, Surgery)

Q.4. Pott's puffy tumour is the:

A. Tuberculosis of spine
B. Bimaleolar ankle fracture
C. Osteomyelitis of skull
D. Bowen's disease

Ans:(C)

- **Pott's spine (Pott's disease)** - ***Tuberculosis of spine.***
- Pott's paraplegia - *Tuberculosis of spine with neurological involvement.*
- Pott's puffy tumour - *Osteomyelitis of skull.*
- #Pott's fracture - *Bimalleolar ankle fracture.*
- **#Cotton's fracture** - ***Trimallelar ankle fracture.***

(Reference: Page No. 174, Maheswari: S. Das, 3rd Edition)

Q.5. Migrating thrombophlebitis seen in:

A. Burger's disease
B. Varicose vein
C. Intra venous infusion
D. Local bacterial infection

Ans: (A)

Migrating thrombophlebitis is seen in:

- Buerger's disease
- Carcinoma of pancreas (Visceral cancer)
- Polycythemia
- Polyarthritis

Varicose vein, Intravenous infusion and Local bacterial infection are the causes of superficial thrombophlebitis.

Try to remember - Homan's sign and Moses sign are seen in deep vein thrombosis.

Q.6. Sister Joseph's nodule is seen:

A. Rheumatoid arthritis
B. Umbilicus
C. Large size condylomata lata
D. Leprosy

Ans: (B)

Sister Joseph's nodule is **secondary carcinoma** of the umbilicus. The **primary neoplasm** is often situated in the **stomach, colon** and **ovary**, but metastasis from breast transmitted along the lymphaticus.

Condylomata lata seen in secondary syphilis.

Try to remember this also:

Adenoma of umbilicus is called as **Rasberry tumour.**

Q.7. Branham's sign is seen in:

A. Aneurysm of aorta
B. Varicose vein
C. AV- Fistula
D. Arterial occlusion

Ans: (C)

Branham's sign also known as Nicoladani's sign. Pressure on the artery proximal to the Fistula causes the swelling to diminish in size, the thrill and bruit to cease, the pulse rate to fall is known as Branham's sign.

AV-Fistula - *congenital* - *Acquired* - Penetrating wound or sharp blow.

AV-Fistula also created surgically for Renal dialysis.

Features:

- Increase pulse rate, Increase cardiac output, Pulse pressure.
- Overgrowth limb (congenital fistula)
- Indolent ulcer
- Left ventricular enlargement.

Q.8. Uvula vesicae is caused by which lobe of prostate:

A. Anterior lobe **B.** Lateral lobe
C. Medial lobe **D.** Posterior lobe

Ans: (C)

- A slight elevation on the trigone immediately posterior to the urethral orifice - produced by median lobe of the prostrate is called as uvula vesicae.
- The lobe for the carcinoma most commonly appears on posterior lobe.
- BPH most commonly appears on median lobe.

(Reference: Page No. 306, BD Chaurasia, 3rd Volume)

Q.9. In pyogenic liver abscess commonest route of spread is:

A. Haematogenous through portal vein
B. Ascending infection through biliary tract
C. Hepatic artery
D. Local spread

Ans: (B)

In pyogenic liver abscess can reach liver in many ways:

a. Along the bile duct (most common route),
b. Via the Portal vein,
c. Via the Hepatic artery,
d. Along the Umbilical vein,
e. By direct extension.

Most common organism: Streptococcus millieri, E-Coli.

Q.10. For breast carcinoma which of the following is best indicator of prognosis:

A. Estrogen receptor status
B. Lymphnode status
C. Metastasis
D. Size of tumor

Ans: (B)

Metastasis to ipsilateral axillary node predicts outcome after surgical treatment more precisely than any other prognostic factor.

Q.11. Not a complication of pseudopancreatic cyst:

A. Hemorrhage into cyst
B. Rupture
C. Malignancy
D. Abscess formation

Ans: (C)

Most common cyst of pancreas: *Pseudocyst.*
The complications of pseudocyst are:

1. Abscess
2. Rupture into peritoneal cavity
3. Haemorrhage
4. Obstuction of Gastro intestinal tract
5. Pseudoaneurysm associated with pseudocyst (Lethal complication).

(Reference: Page No. 995, S. Das, Surgery)

Q.12. Eczema like lesion with frequent bleed around areola is seen in:

A. Eczema
B. Paget's disease
C. Tuberculosis
D. Inflammatory carcinoma

Ans: (B)

Paget's disease associated with intra-duct carcinoma, the tumor cells spreading on the nipple.

Clinical feature

– Red eczamatous like lesion which erodes the nipple

– Eczema usually bilateral, itchy, doesn't destroy the nipple.

Treatment: Simple Mastectomy.

(Reference: Page No. 377, Dutta)

Q.13. Treatment of paralytic ileus include all *except:*

A. Parasympathomimetics

B. Nasogastric aspirate

C. Electrolyte correction

D. Symphatomimetics

Ans: (D)

Paralytic is a dynamic intestinal obstruction.

Important sign:

- Distension of abdomen, absent bowel sound and failure to pass flatus.
- Most common cause are post operative paralytic ileus.

Treatment:

- ➢ Nasogastric suction,
- ➢ Intravenous fluid administration,
- ➢ Correction of Elecrolyte Imbalance (Hypokalemia),
- ➢ Parasympathomimetics are used (Neostigmine).

(Reference: Page No. 984, S.Das 3rd Edition)

Q.14. Acute pancreatic causes all *except:*

A. Fat necrosis

B. Hypercalcemia

C. Increased amylase

D. Increased lipase.

Ans: (B)

- Hypocalcemia is the feature of acute pancreatitis.
- Increased serum lipase is diagnostic of acute pancreatitis moreover the duration of hyperlipasemia often exceeds that of Hyperamylasemia.
- C.T.Scan in the investigation of choice.

SURGERY

The complaints of acute pancreatitis are:

1. Shock and Acute renal failure.
2. Hyperglycemia, Hypocalcemia, Hypoxia.
3. Pancreatic abscess, Pseudocyst and Obstructions.

Q.15. Grey turner sign is seen in:

A. Acute cholecystitis
B. Acute pancreatitis
C. Acute appendicitis
D. Tumor of spleen

Ans: (B)

Grey turner sign: Discolouration of yellowish brown due to ecchymosis of extravasated blood in the loin in acute haemorrhagic pancreatitis.

Collen sign: Discoloration of periumbilical region in acute **hemorrhagic pancreatitis.**

(Reference: Page No. 934, S. Das 3rd edition)

Q.16. A 45-year-man complain of vomiting with food mass taken days before, foul smelling breath. Occasional dysphagia to solid food. What is the diagnosis?

A. Zenker's diverticulum
B. Achalasia
C. Diabetic gastro paresis
D. Scleroderma

Ans: (A)

- *Zenker's diverticulum* (also known as pharyngoesophageal diverticula).
- It is the most common esophageal diverticula.
- *Age:* patient older than 60 years.
- *Site:* Diverticulum characteristically arises within the inferior pharyngeal constrictor between the oblique fibres and horizontal fibres, (at killians triangle).
- Zenker's diverticulum is a **pulsion** diverticulum.
- *Symptoms:* Dysphagia (Particularly for solid foods) Regurgitation of food. Halitosis, Voice change, Retro sternal pain and Respiratory obstruction.

- Most common complication of Zenker's diverticulum is Lung abscess due to Aspiration.

(Reference: Page No. 715, Sabiston 16th Edition)

Q.17. Most common type of Basal cell carcinoma:

A. Cystic type
B. Morphea type
C. Noduloulcerative type
D. Pigmented type

Ans: (C)

- Basal cell carcinoma is commonest form of skin cancer.
- Called as **Rodent ulcer.**
- Arises from basal cell layer of epidermis.
- It is locally invasive, it does not spreads through Lymphatics or blood stream.
- Most common site, **Inner canthus of eye.**
- Most common type **Noduloulcerative type**.
- Most aggressive and high recurrence in morphea type.
- *Treatment:* **Excision** with healthy margin. It is good **radiosensitive tumour** also.

SURGERY

Q.18. Collar - Stud abscess is seen in:

A. Actinomycosis
B. Tuberculosis
C. Syphilis
D. Sarcoidosis

Ans: (B)

- Collar - Stud abscess - It is bi-locular abscess with one locule deep to deep fascia and another locule in superficial fascia.
- They inter communicate through perforation in deep fascia.

2 types:

Pyogenic → More often in **Palmar fascia.**
Tuberculous → More often in **neck.**

Cold abscesses:

It is not hot and red as **Pyogenic abscesses.**

Seen in tuberculosis, Actinomycosis, Gumma degeneration, Leprosy.

(Reference: Page No. 635, S. Das 3rd Edition)

Q.19. Spigelian hernia is seen in:

A. Lumbar triangle

B. Supra umbilical region

C. Arcuate line

D. Paraumbilical region

Ans: (C)

- Spegelian hernia is an Interparietal hernia, that occurs at the level of Arcuate line, that is subumbilical region.
- It is situated beneath Internal oblique, or between the Internal and external oblique muscles.
- *Diagnosis:* CT or USG.
- *Para - umbilical hernia:* Protrusion through linea alba, just above or below the umblicus.

Q.20. Calculus is most common in which salivary gland:

A. Sublingual **B.** Parotid

C. Submandibular **D.** Sublingual

Ans: (C)

- *Eighty* percent of all salivary gland stones occur in the submandibular gland, 10% occur in the parotid, 7% in the sublingual and remainder occurs in minor salivary glands.
- *Eight* percent of submandibular stones are Radioopaque.
- Majority of parotid gland stones are **radiolucent.**

Remember

- Most common benign salivary gland tumours - ***Plemorphic adenoma.***
- Most common malignant salivary gland tumour - ***Mucoepidermoid carcinoma.***
- The parotid gland tumour which spreads through neural sheath - ***Adenoid cystic carcinoma.***

Q.21. Most common organ ruptures in blunt trauma of abdomen:

A. Diaphragm

B. Liver

C. Spleen

D. Kidney

Ans: (C)

Splenic ruptures should be suspected after any trauma, particularly any direct injury to left upper quadrant from any angle.

(Reference: Page No. 955, Bailey and love, 23rd Edition. Page No. 896, S. Das Textbook of Surgery)

Q.22. Hirshprung's disease most commonly involves:

A. Jejunum

B. Illeo-colic junctions

C. Rectosigmoid junctions

D. Upper sigmoid part

Ans: (C)

- In about two third of patients the rectum and lower part of sigmoid colon are involved, but involvement short segments of the lower rectum or the whole intestinal tract have been described.
- Tooth paste like stool is the classical finding.
- Common complications are enterocolitis and perforation of bowel.

(Reference: Page No. 1027, Bailey and Love, 23rd Edition)

Q.23. Dumping syndrome is characterized by all *except:*

A. Hyperglycemia

B. Tremor

C. Tachycardia

D. Diarrhoea

Ans: (A)

➢ Dumping syndrome - *following gastrectomy or vagotomy.*

- Early and late dumping - *different etilogies but common features of rapid gastric emptying.*
  - *Early dumping symptoms:* Epigastric fullness, Sweating, Light headedness, Tachycardia, Colic, diarrhoea.
  - *Late dumping symptoms:* you can see Reactive Hypoglycemia not a hyperglycemia.

(Reference: Page No. 913, Bailey and Love)

Q.24. All are complication of Crohn's disease *except:*

A. Sclerosing cholangitis
B. Intestinal fistulas
C. Intestinal stricture
D. Toxic megacolon

Ans: (D)

	Ulcerative colitis	Crohn's disease
Rectal involvement	M/c >90%	*Ileocaecal junction - most common - Rectal spare in 50%*
Lesions	**Continuous** *where mouth to anus*	*Skip lesion from any*
Inflammation	**Mucosal and submucosal**	*Transmural*
Barium meal features	- **Pipe stem colon** - Loss of Haustrations - **Pseudopolyposis**	*- String sign of kantor* *- Cobble stone appearance* *- Lead pipe Fibrous thickening*
Complications *and obstruction*	**Not seen**	*- Intestinal strictures* *- Intestinal fistula* *- Fissures* *- Perianal abscess* *- Fistulas*
Extra intestinal manifestations		
Sclerosing pericholangitis	**Common**	*Rare*
Uveitis and Arthritis	**Common**	*Common*
Pyoderma gangrenosum	**Rare**	*Not seen*
Carcinoma	**10%**	*Very rare*
Granulomas	**Not seen**	*Common*

Toxic megacolon is seen in ulcerative colitis.

Q.25. Best marker to assess prognosis after colon surgery:

A. CA-125 **B.** CEA

C. CA- 15.3 **D.** PSA

Ans: (B)

List of important markers:

- Medullary carcinoma of thyroid - *Calcitonin, Neuron specific enolase*
- Carcinoid - *5-HIAA*
- Stomach - *Gastrin*
- Pituitary - *ACTH*
- Bone - *Alkaline phosphate*
- Multiple myeloma - *Ben Jone protein*
- Prostate - *PSA, Prostatic acid phosphate*
- Liver - *AFP, Carcino embryonic antigen (CEA)*
- Ovary - *CA-125, Beta-HCG*
- Breast - *CA-15.3,*
- Testicle - *AFP, Beta HCG, LDH*
- Colon—*CEA.*

Q.26. Amylase is increased in all *except:*

A. Acute appendicitis

B. Acute pancreatitis

C. Duodenal perforation

D. Intestinal obstruction

Ans: (A)

Pancreatic disease causing elevated amylase level:

- Acute pancreatitis
- Pancreatic abscess
- Pancreatic pseudocyst
- Complication of pancreatitis

Some important non-pancreatic disorders are:

- Mumps
- Pregnancy
- Perforation peptic ulcer
- Ruptured ectopic pregnancy
- Intestinal obstruction or infarction
- Cholecystitis
- Diabetic ketoacidosis
- Burn

Q.27. GERD (Gastro Esophageal Reflux Disease) is Predisposed by:

A. Smoking

B. Defective gastric emptying

C. Truncal vagotomy

D. All

Ans: (D)

GERD predisposing factors:

1. Dietary factors (alcohol, smoking, chocolate, fat foods)
2. Defective esophageal clearance
3. Delayed gastric emptying
4. Increasing Intra abdominal pressure

GERD is mainly due to function loss of competence of lower esophageal sphincter.

(Reference: Page No. 776, Davidson's 16th Edition)

Q.28. Chronic cholecystitis is associated with all ***except:***

A. Usually palpable

B. Common in women

C. Associated with Gallbladder stones

D. Rokitansky-Aschoff sinuses

Ans: (A)

- Gallbladder is not palpable, there is usually right upper quadrant tenderness, and no muscle guarding is there.
- Rokitansky-Aschoff sinuses are found in 90% case chronic cholecystitis.
- Gallbladder stones are most commonly associated with chronic cholecystitis.
- Gallbladder stones are most commonly seen in Fatty, Fertile, Flatulent, Females of fifty.

(Reference:Page No. 906, S.Das-3rd Edition)

Q.29. All the following Lymphnodes involved in breast carcinoma ***except:***

A. Axillary node

B. Pretracheal node

C. Parasternal node

D. Supraclavicular node

Ans: (B)

The lymphnodes involved in breast carcinoma are axillary, Internal mammary, intraclavicular, Supraclavicular and Parasternal node.

Q.30. All are precancerous state of penis *except:*

A. Hypospadias

B. Chronic balanoposthitis

C. Hpv infection

D. Paget's disease of penis

Ans: (A)

The precancerous states are:

- Genital warts (Hpv infection)
- Paget's disease of penis
- Balanitis xerotica obliterans
- Chronic balanoposthitis
- Most common type of carcinoma in penis → *squamous cell carcinoma.*
- Most common site → *Origin is Glans penis.*
- Circumcision after birth decreases the risk of carcinoma penis.

Q.31. Perforation of typhoid ulcer usually occurs during ________ week:

A. 1st week **B.** 2nd week

C. 3rd week **D.** 4th week

Ans: (C)

- Typhoid is mainly medical disease, which caused by *salmonella typhi.*
- In this disease there is hyperplasia, Ulceration of payer's patches of the intestine which present antimesenteric border of ilium, Mesenteric lymphadenopathy.
- Confirmation diagnosis is obtained by culturing S.Typhi from blood or feaces or by finding a high titre of agglutinins against the O and H antigens of the organism.
- Complication of the disease with which the surgeon concerned with:
  - Intestinal haemorrhage (10-20% cases)
  - Intestinal perforation (2% cases) which is during 3rd week.

- Perforation occurs through ulcerated Payer's patches in the **Terminal Ileum.**
- It must be remembered that these ulcers are **Longitudinal**.

Remember:

Tubercular ulcer, which are **transverse** because it follows lymphatic channel.

But amoebic ulcers are **flask** shaped.

- Paralytic Ileus - Most common complication, It is associated with distension of abdomen.
  Treatment: Conservative.
- Cholecystitis - When patient become carrier.
- Joints → Mild effusion.
- Bones → Makes typhoid osteomyelitis (Rarely)
- Genitourinary complication - Typhoid pyelitis, Cystitis, Epidermo-orchitis.

(Reference: P. No. 973, S. Das - 3rd Edition)

Q.32. Not a malignant change in pleomorphic adenoma:

A. Facial nerve palsy

B. Trismus

C. Pain

D. Cervical lymphnode enlargement

Ans: (B)

Pleomorphic adenoma is the most common Benign Tumor of salivary gland. In the parotid gland the commonest location is the **tail of the gland.**

Symptom: The patient complain of painless swelling of the side of the face.

Examination:

- **Shape** - The tumour tends to be **Round** or **Oval** when it is small.
- **Surface** - the surface is **smooth.**
- **Edge** - The margins are **quite distinct**.
- **Fixing** - It is neither adherent to the skin nor the masseter muscle.
- **Involvement of facial nerve** - Even when the Tumor is huge the facial nerve is not involved and remains free. Involvement of facial nerve indicated by paralysis of

SURGERY

involved Facial muscles. Indicates carcinomatous change.

- **Cervical lymphnode** - Though rare yet malignant transformation of this tumor may occur in 3-5% of cases. Malignant transformation is apprehended when the tumor:
  - Becomes painful.
  - Starts growing rapidly.
  - Feels stony hard.
  - Gets fixed to the masseter deeply or to the skin superficially.
  - Involves facial nerve is an important feature of malignancy.
  - Cervical lymphnode enlargement.
  - Causes restriction of movement of the jaw.

Important:

Superficial parotidectomy is the treatment of choice for Pleomorphic adenoma. This operation is also known as *Patey's operation.*

Trismus in para pharyngeal abscess is due to spasm of *Medial pterygoid muscle.*

SURGERY

Q.33. The mass of 15 cm away from the anal orifice, the treatment of choice is:

A. Colonoscopic removal
B. Hartman's operation
C. Anterior resection
D Abdomino perineal resection

Ans: (C)

Rectum is divided into 3 parts:
Proximal third of rectum
Middle third of rectum
Lower third of rectum

Operation of rectum are:

There are numerous procedures for treating rectal carcinoma. out of these, most commonly asked in exams are:

1. Anterior resection
2. Abdomino perineal resection
3. Hartman's procedure

- **Anterior resection** is a sphincter saving procedure and it is done for the carcinoma in the proximal third of the rectum and middle third of rectum. It is not done for the carcinoma of rectum which are 7cm from anal verge.
- Abdomino perineal resection - It is the treatment of the choice of carcinoma of rectum which are within the 7 cm from anal verge. Here sphincter is sacrificed and permanent colostomy is performed.

Note:

If you get the choice that carcinoma is 7 cm from dentate line then the treatment of choice will be anterior resection because you have to add 2.5 cm because dentate line is 2.5 cm from anal verge. so the length will be 7 + 2.5 = 9.5 cm. So the carcinoma of the rectum is 9 cm from the anal verge. Treatment of choice will be antérior resection.

(Reference: P. No. 1067, S. Das 3rd Edition)

Q.34. Complications of Duodenal ulcer, all *except:*

A. Malignancy **B.** Perforation
C. Bleeding **D.** Obstruction.

Ans: (A)

Duodenal ulcer almost never changes to Malignancy. Incidence of Malignant change in gastric ulcer is not very definitely know ulcer near the greater curvature and near the lesser curvature below the angulus are more prone to malignant change.

The common complication of peptic ulcer is:

1. Bleeding
2. Stenosis
3. Perforation
4. Gastric outlet obstruction.

Remember

The most common site of benign peptic ulcer is → lesser curvature near incisura Angularis.
The most common site of duodenal ulcer is → 1st part of duodenum.

(Reference: Page No. 850 S. Das 3rd Edition)

SURGERY

SEVENTEEN

Obstetrics & Gynaecology

Q.1. A patient soon after 3rd stage of labour, placenta came out fully, but there is heavy bleed, the Rx is:

A. IVF

B. Check for placenta in uterus

C. Check for Laceration of Labia

D. Massage and oxytocin

Ans: (D)

- Here in this case there is no placenta left inside the uterus, they had clearly mentioned the placenta fully came out.
- So the best choice is to **palpate the fundus, massage and oxytocin**

(Reference: P.No 413, Dutta's Text of Obs)

Q.2. Gold standard for conforming the diagnosis of PID:

A. USG

B. Laparoscopy

C. Blood leucocyte count

D. Antichalmydial Ab.

Ans: (B)

In acute PID laparoscopy is an excellent means of obtaining cultures directly from the tube. Laparoscopy is still considered the gold standard for conforming the diagnosis of PID, because it not only allows direct inspection of Fallopian tubes and surrounding pelvic anatomy but also enables microbiologic sampling from the upper genital tract (e.g. fallopian tube, ovary and peritoneal fluid).

(Reference: Telinde's Operative Gynaecology 9th Edition. Page No. 679, Shaw's Textbook of Operative Gynae 6th Edition. P. No. 164)

Q.3. Bacterial vaginosis can cause all *except:*

A. Abruptio placenta
B. Endometritis
C. Chorioamnionitis
D. Pre-term labour

Ans: (A)

Bacterial vaginosis is nothing but gardenella vaginosis.

It is termed as vaginosis because a patient is associated with alteration in normal vaginal flora. There is considerable decrease in no. of bacilli with 100 fold growth of other bacteria.

Characteristics of vaginal discharge:

1. White milky discharge.
2. Ph > 4.5.
3. Fishy odour.
4. Clue cells and gardnella are seen.

The infection can cause PID, chroioamnionitis, premature rupture of membrane, preterm labour.

Rx. DOC - *Metronidazole*

(Reference: 30, Shaw's 13th Edition)

Q.4. Down's syndrome is diagnosed in a pregnant women by all *except:*

A. Decreased AFP
B. Increased HCG
C. Decreased HCG
D. Estriol

Ans: (C)

Triple test is combined biochemical test usually done at 15-18 weeks includes

a. MSAFP (Maternal serum α-feto protein) is decreased
b. HCG is increased
c. UE (unconjugated oestriol) is decreased

It is used for detection of down syndrome. Triple test gives risk ratio (1:250) for confirmation of diagnosis by amniocentesis.

Test available for detection of down syndrome are:

1. Noninvasive test
2. Invasive test

NONINVASIVE TEST

- Maternal serum analysis
- Maternal urinary analysis
- Ultrasonography

INVASIVE TEST

- Chronic villous sampling (9-12 weeks)
- Amniocentesis (15-18 weeks)

Noninvasive test are done when the pregnancy are not at risk.

Invasive test are done when the pregnancy is at risk.

The Risk factors are:

- Advanced maternal age > 35 yrs (Risk 1-10%)
- Parent with a balanced translocation (Risk 3-20%)
- Previous child with down syndrome (1%)

(Reference: Dutta 5th Edition P. No. 112)

Q.5. In vagina, the type of epithelium is:

A. Columnar

B. Non-keratinised stratified squamous

C. Keratinised squamous

D. Cuboidal

Ans: (B)

To remember:

Epithelial lining of:

Vagina - *Non keratinised stratified squamous*

Cervix - *Columnar*

Uterus - *Ciliated columnar*

Urinary bladder - *Transitional*

Oral cavity - *Non keratinised stratified squamous*
Tonsil - *Non keratinised stratified squamous*
Bartholin duct - *Serous*
PCT - *Broad based columnar cell.*
DCT - *Cuboidal epithelium*

Loop of Henle

Descending

Upper part - *Columnar epithelium*
Lower part - *Squamous epithelium*

Ascending

Lower part - *Squamous epithelium*
Upper part - *Cuboidal epithelium*

Q.6. Exact no. of weeks between LMP and EDD:

A. 37 weeks
B. 38 weeks
C. 39 weeks
D. 40 weeks

Ans: (D)

Expected date of delivery is calculated by using Naegle's formula by adding 9 calendar month and 7 days from the first day of last menstruation (28 days cycle) period.

Q.7. A composite graphical record of cervical dilation and descent of head against duration of labour in hours known as:

A. Apgar score
B. Partogram
C. Bishop's score
D. Pearl index

Ans: (B)

Apgar score: *It is related to the status of oxygenation of the fetus at or immediately after birth. Long-term neurological correlation is obtained at the 5 minute score which is of more value. In cases where the score remains significantly depressed at 5 minutes. It should be evaluated again after 15 minutes. This scoring is done in a newborn baby at 1 minute,*

5 minutes and 15 minutes. In this scoring we see respiratory effort, Heart rate, Muscle tone, Reflex irritability and Colour.

- Total apgar score is 10
- No depression is 7-10
- Mild depression is 4-6
- Severe depression is 0-3

Partogram: *It is a composite graphical record of cervical dilation and descent of head against duration of labour in hours.*

The component of a partograph are:

- *Patient identification*
- *Time*
- *Fetal heat rate*
- *State of membranes and colour of liquor*
- *Cervical dilatation and descent of the head*
- *Uterine contractions*
- *Drugs and fluids*
- *Blood pressure at every 2 hours and pulse at every 30 minutes*
- *Oxytosin*
- *Urine analysis*
- *Temperature record*

Bishops score: *Bishop's pre-induction cervical scoring system includes parameters like:*

- *Dilatation of cervix*
- *Cervical length of cervix*
- *Consistency of cervix*
- *Position of cervix*
- *Station of head*

Total score = 13

Favourable score = 6-13

Unfavourable score = 0-5

Pearl index: *The failure rate of any contraceptive is calculated in terms of pregnancy rate per hundred women years of use. It is calculated according to the following formula:*

- Pregnancy failure rate = Number of accidental pregnancies × 1200/Number of patients observed × Months of use.

- When the pregnancy rate is below 10, the effectiveness of the particular method is considered to be high. If it is more than 20, it is said to be low.
- Failure rate of contraceptive methods in first 12 months of use per 100 women are:
  - ➢ *Tuberectomy = 0.5*
  - ➢ *Vasectomy = 0.15*
  - ➢ *Norplant = 0.1*
  - ➢ *DMPA and NET injectables = 0.3*
  - ➢ *Progestin only pill = 1*
  - ➢ *Combined oral pill = 0.1*
  - ➢ *IUCD = 0.5-2*
  - ➢ *Diaphragm = 20*
  - ➢ *Condom (male) = 14*
  - ➢ *Lactational amenorrhoea = 2*
  - ➢ *Coitus interruptus = 19*
  - ➢ *Rhythm = 24*
  - ➢ *No method = 80*

(Reference: Page Nos. 471, 522, 529, 531, D.C. Dutta Obstetrics - 6th Edition)

Q.8. Colposcopy used to visualize:

A. Cervix
B. Uterus
C. Fallopian tube
D. All of the above

Ans: (A)

- *Cervix is visualized by* ***colposcopy with*** **Magnification to 40 times.**
- **Colposcopy** directed biopsy is the best one when the lesion is not clinically detected.
- Fallopian tube is visualized by **salpingoscopy (falloposcopy)**, Mainly used selection of patients for IVF (In Vitro Fertilization).
- *Uterus is visualized by* ***Hysteroscopy***, used in unresponsive uterine bleeding, Uterine Synechiae, Congenital uterine septum, Missing IUD threads, etc.
- ***Colpomicroscopy*** *is used to see the structures at cellular level (100 to 300 times magnification).*

OBS. & GYNAE.

- **Culdoscopy** - Optical instrument to visualize the pelvic structure, through an incision in the pouch of Douglas.

Q.9. LH: FSH ratio increased in:

A. Menopause
B. PCOD
C. Testicular feminization
D. Turners syndrome

Ans: (B)

LH: FSH ratio is > 3:1 in PCOD (LH increased, FSH decreased)

PCOD is also known as Stein Leventhal syndrome

Characteristic features:

- *Hirsutism*
- *Obesity*
- *Oligomenorrhoea or Amenorrhoea*
- *Infertility*

M/c cause of hirsutism and virilising syndrome in young women.

Lab finding

- Decreased FSH and progesterone (may be absent)
- No ovulation - no progesterone
- USG - Necklace appearance of ovaries
- *DOC:* **Clomiphene citrate**
- Turner's syndrome - Testicular feminization, menopause both LH and FSH are increased.

Q.10. M/c position in vertex presentation:

A. LOA **B.** ROA
C. LOP **D.** ROP

Ans: (A)

Vertex occupying the left anterior quadrant of the pelvis is the commonest one and called as left occipito anterior.

Presentation	*Diameter of Engagement*
Vertex	Sub-occipito Bregmatic
Brow	Vertico mental
Face	Submento-Bregmatic
Breech	Bi-ischial

OBS. & GYNAE.

Shoulder Bi-acromial

M/c - *presentation is cephalic (96.5%)*

M/c - *presenting part of cephalic -vertex (96%)*

M/c - *lie-longitudinal lie (99.5%)*

(Reference: Page No. 77, Dutta)

Q.11. Investigation to be done in a girl presenting with delayed puberty:

A. USG pelvis **B.** FSH

C. Karyotyping **D.** All above

Ans: (D)

Here they didn't ask anything specifically. So you have to rule out all the possible methods.

Q.12. Advantage of median episiotomy over mediolateral are all *except:*

A. Hemorrhage is less

B. Healing is good

C. Extension of incision

D. Repair is easy

Ans: (C)

- You can't extend the Incision as it may involve the rectum. It is the major disadvantage of median episiotomy.
- To extent the incision—mediolateral episiotomy is relatively safer, it is used commonly, but Dyspareunia is comparatively more.
- The other two type's episiotomy- lateral and J shaped.
- Relative merits and demerits of median and mediolateral episiotomy:

Merits of median episiotomy:

- ➢ *The muscles are not cut.*
- ➢ *Blood loss is least.*
- ➢ *Repair is easy.*
- ➢ *Post operative comfort is maximum.*
- ➢ *Healing is superior.*
- ➢ *Wound disruption is rare.*
- ➢ *Dyspareunia is rare.*

Demerits of median episiotomy:

- *Extension, if occurs, may involve the rectum.*
- *Not suitable for manipulative delivery or in abnormal presentation or position. As such, its use is selective.*

Merits of mediolateral episiotomy:

- *Relative safety from rectal involvement from extension.*
- *If necessary, the incision can be extended.*

Demerits of mediolateral episiotomy:

- *Apposition of the tissue is not so good.*
- *Blood loss is little more.*
- *Post operative discomfort is more.*
- *Relative increased incidence of wound disruption.*
- *Dyspareunia is comparatively more.*

(Reference: P. No. 568 Dutta)

Q.13. Bishop scoring system measures:

A. Cervical changes during delivery
B. To record the progress of labour
C. Intrauterine fetal well being.
D. For the uterine contraction

Ans: (A)

Follow the explanation of question no. 7 of obstetrics and gynaecology.

Q.14. Ovulation coincides with:

A. FSH surge
B. LH surge
C. Peak of progesterone
D. Peak of oestrogen

Ans: (B)

- Ovulation approximately occurs at 16-24 hrs after the LH surge
- The rupture of graffian follicule due to contraction of micro muscle present over Theca externa. These contraction brought by prostaglandin secreted under the influence of LH.

- The ovulation and maturation can be studied by serial USG.

(Reference: Page No. 20, OBS Dutta/Page No. 28 - Shaw Gynaecology)

Q.15. Painless heavy bleed is seen in:

A. Ectopic pregnancy
B. Abruptio placenta
C. Placenta previa
D. Abortion

Ans: (C)

Placenta previa—It is when the placenta implanted partially or completely over the lower uterine segment

1. **Features**—*painless, causeless, recurrent bleeding, fresh bleed, placenta in lower segment/low lying.*
2. Uterus soft and relaxed.
3. **Diagnosed by:** *USG, FHS usually present.*
4. **Rx:** *PV examination is delayed upto 37 wk to avoid premature labour, PV should be performed in OT room.*

Abruptio placenta

- Painful, continuous bleeding with toxaemic features.
- Concealed bleed (may be mixed)
- Sign of fetal distress and shock
- Associated with pre-eclampsia
- Placenta in upper segment
- Uterus is tense, tender and light
- FHS usually be absent
- Diagnosed clinically

Rx:

Correction of hypovolumic shock - 1st priority. *Give dexamethasone and deliver the baby by induction.*

Q.16. Most common site of ectopic pregnancy:

A. Isthmus **B.** Fimbriae
C. Interstitium **D.** Ampulla of tube

Ans: (D)

- Most common site of ectopic pregnancy is ampullary part of fallopian tube.
- Fallopian tube is 10 cm long which has 4 parts.
  - *Interstitial - narrowest part of fallopian tube*
  - *Isthmus*
  - *Ampulla - widest part*
  - *Fimbria*
- Most common cause of ectopic pregnancy is Pelvic inflammatory disease (6 - 10 fold).
- The longest survival in ectopic pregnancy of fallopian tube is in the **Isthmus.**

(Reference: D.C. Dutta Page No. 179)

Q.17. 43 years lady complain of prolonged and heavy bleed through vagina. On examination endometrial hyperplasia, which is not atypical? What is the treatment?

A. Hysterectomy
B. Progestins
C. Radio therapy
D. OCPs

Ans: (B)

- Common causes of menorrhagia are DUB or chronic pelvic infection.
- Common causes of contact bleeding are carcinoma cervix, cervical mucous polyp and vascular erosion.
- The endometrial pattern in DUB is secretary in 60% and hyper plastic in about 30%.
- There is no hormone therapy in postmenopausal DUB.
- In premenopausal (>40 years) patient absence of any +ve finding, where bleeding continues even after uterine curettage, *cyclic progestogen* therapy may be employed judiciously.
- If in premenopausal patients have *adenomatous* or *atypical endometrial hyperplasia* requires *hysterectomy.*

- In reproductive period (20-40 years), if patients have irregular excessive cycle, we have to do investigation by USG (TVS).

(Reference: Dutta Gyne, 3rd Edition. Page-No. 184.)

Q.18. The complication of hydramnios are all *except:*

A. Hemorrhage
B. Obstructed labour
C. Uterine inertia
D. Prematurity

Ans: (B)

Polyhydramnios is a state where liquor amniotic fluid exceeds 2000 ml.

Most common cause of polyhydraminosis are:

- Fetal anomalies – *anencephaly*
  – open spina bifida
  – GIT Atresia
  – hydrops fetalis
- Placenta – *chorioangioma*
- Multiple pregnancy
- Maternal – Diabetes

Complications:

Maternal during pregnancy:

- Pre eclampsia
- Malpresentation
- Premature rupture of membrane
- Hemorrhage

Maternal during labour:

- Early rupture of membrane
- Cord prolapse
- Uterine inertia.
- Retained placenta
- Postpartum hemorrhage

Fetal:

↑ perinatal mortality (death are due to prematurity and congenital abnormality

(Reference: Dutta Obs, 6rd Edition, Page No. 216)

EIGHTEEN

Paediatrics

Q.1. 4-hour fluid requirement of a baby of 8 kg with severe dehydration:

A. 1000 ml

B. 800 ml

C. 600 ml

D. 500 ml

Ans: (C)

If the weight of child is known the amount of ORS solution required for rehydration during the first four hours may be calculated by setting the deficit at approximately **75 ml/kg**. If the child's weight is not known the approximate deficit may be determined on the basis of age.

So, weight of child is 8 kg.

Setting the deficit of approximately - 75 ml/kg

Then $8 \times 75 = 600$ ml

(Reference: Page No. 180, Table, Park - 18th Edition)

Q.2. Delayed bone age is due to:

A. Hyperthyroidism

B. Hypothyroidism

C. Congenital adrenal hyperplasia

D. Cushing syndrome

Ans: (B)

- When bone age (Epiphyseal development) is less than the chronological age. Then it is known as **delayed bone age.**
- **Markedly delayed**: *Hypothyroidism, Hypopitutrism.*
- **Moderately delayed**: *Malnutrition, Chronic infection.*
- **Mild delay:** *Constitutional delay.*

Boneage is in advance of the heightage

- Familial short stature
- Down syndrome
- Turner syndrome
- Chondrodystrophies
- Intrauterine infection
- Storage disorders

Boneage is an advance chronologic age

- Precocious puberty
- Thyrotoxicosis

(Reference: Page No: 52. O.P. Ghai)

Q.3. Physiological jaundice in a term baby is maximum at:

A. 5 days **B.** 6 days
C. 7 days **D.** 9 days

Ans: (A)

Physiological Jaundice:

- Appears after 24 hours
- Intensifies in 5 days in term baby and 7 days in preterm infant (12-15 mg/dl)
- Total bilirubin <15 mg/dl
- After two weeks clinically not detachable, adult values are attained

Pathological Jaundice:

- Pathologic Jaundice appears in the first 24 hours
- Total bilirubin >15 mg/dl (Hyperbilirubinemia)
- Direct bilirubin >2.0 mg/dl
- Persist more than 14 days.

(Reference: Page No. 171, OP.Ghai - 6th Edition)

Q.4. Enuresis is normal until:

A. 1½ years **B.** 2½ years
C. 4 years **D.** 5 years

Ans: (D)

Enuresis is defined as normal nearly complete evacuation of the bladder at a wrong place and time atleast twice a month after the **Fifth** year of life.

(Reference: Page No. 61, O.P.Ghai)

Q.5. Single oral dose for vitamin D prophylaxis:

A. 25000 IU
B. 50000 IU
C. 100000 IU
D. 200000 IU

Ans: (C)

Daily requirements:
Adult - *2.5 mcg (100 IU)*
Infants and children - *5.0 mcg (200 IU)*
Pregnancy and Lactation - *10.0 mcg (400 IU)*
(One IU of Vitamin D is 0.025mg of Calciferol)
For management of Rickets - *administration of 15000 mg or 600000 IU of Vitamin D3 orally or IM induces rapid healing.*

Q.6. For vesico ureteric reflex investigation of choice is:

A. X-Ray
B. MCU
C. CT-Scan
D. Antegrade orogram

Ans: (B)

VUR - refers to retrograde flow of urine from the bladder to the **Upper urinary tract.**
Two techniques commonly used to detect VUR, The radio contrast MCU is most commonly used. Since in addition to showing VUR, it provides excellent anatomical details.
Isotope Radionuclide Cystography is more **Sensitive:** For detecting VUR and causes Less radiation exposure but provides less anatomical details. So, MCV is the investigation of choice for VUR. But **Isotope Radionuclide Cystography** is more sensitive.

(Reference: Page No: 457, OP.Ghai - 6th Edition)

Q.7. Investigation of choice to diagnose Hirchsprung's disease is:

A. Rectal manometry
B. Barium enema
C. Rectal biopsy
D. Laparotomy

Ans: (C)

Definitive diagnosis of Hirschprung's disease is made by:

- **Rectal biopsy** - Absence of ganglion cells in Meissner's plexus, myenteric plexus and Hypertrophy of nerve trunks.
- **Manometric study** - Show a failure of relaxation of internal sphincter following rectal distention. It is used as screening test.
- **Barium enema** also helpful in diagnosis, but not Investigation of choice.

(Reference: CSTD 10th Edition)

Q.8. 100% oxygen improves cyanosis in all *except:*

A. Tetralogy of fallot
B. Bronchial asthma
C. Eosinophilic pneumonia
D. Interstitial lung disease

Ans: (B)

O2 therapy is helpful in V/Q Mismatch.

- Airway disease (Asthma COPD)
- Interstitial lung disease
- Alveolar disease
- Pulmonary vascular disease.

O2 therapy is not helpful.

- Alveolar collapse (Atelectasis)
- Intra-alveolar filling - (Pneumonia, Pulmonary edema)
- Intracardiac shunt (R-L shunt)
- Vascular shunt within lungs.

(Reference: Harrison 16th Edition, Page No. 1504)

Q.9. Wide and Split S_2 occurs in:

A. Coarctation of Aorta
B. VSD
C. ASD
D. MS

Ans: (C)

Wide fixed splitting of S_2 with ejection systolic murmur in left 2nd intercostals space points towards the diagnosis of Arterial septal defect.

Also know:

Paradoxical reverse splitting is seen in complete left bundle branch block, Right ventricular pacemaker.

Most common type of ASD - **Ostium Secundum**

(Reference: O.P.GHAI. 5th Edition, Page No. 296 & 297)

Q.10. Prophylaxis to a child with RHD should be given minimum till:

A. Atleast 5 years after onset
B. Life long
C. Till 17 years
D. Till 21 years

Ans: (A)

- There is controversy over this question. Davidson says that attacks of rheumatic fever are unusual after the age of 21 at which age treatment may be stopped.
- Harrison say, that the risk of recurrence of RF is highest during the first 5 years after the attack secondary prophylaxis is always given for at least this period.
- This is a controversial question. We will go with Harrison.
- **Some Important points:**
  Endocarditis is unusual in sites with a small pressure gradient as in ASD. VSD is most common congenital lesion to be complicated by infective endocarditis. Most common valve involved in IV drug abusers is tricuspid valve.

PAEDIATRICS

NINETEEN

PSM

Q.1. Most important indicator of protein efficacy:

A. Biological value
B. Net protein utilization
C. Amino acid score
D. Protein energy ratio

Ans: (B)

- The NPU of a protein is the proportion of ingested nitrogen that is retained in the body under specified conditions. NPU is a combined measure of digestibility and the efficiency of utilization of the absorbed amino acids.
- Recommended protein intake for Indian reference adult male is 60 g/day.
- Recommended protein intake for Indian reference woman is 50 g/day.
- Recommended protein intake for Indian reference pregnant woman is 65 g/day.
- Recommended protein intake for Indian reference lactating woman is 75 g/day.

(Reference: Ghai, Page No. 94 and Park 18th Edition Page No. 459)
(Reference Protein is EGG)

Q.2. Dietary fibers rich in:

A. Polysaccharide
B. Monosaccharide
C. Non starch polysaccharide
D. None of the above.

Ans: (C)

- A dietary fiber rich in mainly non starch polysaccharide is a physiologically important component of the diet. It is found in vegetables fruits and grains. They cannot be digested by animals own digestive enzymes Eg: *Cellulose, hemicellulose, pectins, gums legnins and pentosans.*

- The fibers absorb water and this increased the bulk of stool and helps to reduce constipation by increasing the transit time.
- Fiber may also have a role in weight reduction. The cholesterol lowering effect of certain types of dietary fibers appears firmly established.

(Reference: 18th Edition Park, Page No. 442)

Q.3. Saturated fatty acids maximum in:

A. Coconut oil **B.** Butter
C. Margarine **D.** Palm oil

Ans: (A)

Fatty Acids (FA): Fats yield fatty acid and glycerol on hydrolysis. Fatty acids are divided into saturated fatty acids such as lauric, palmitic , stearic acids and polyunsaturated fatty acids (PUFA) e.g. *Linoleic Acids and Linolenic Acid.* The polyunsaturated fatty acids are mostly found in vegetables oils and the saturated fatty acids are found mainly in animal fats. However there are exceptions as for example. Coconut and palm oils although they are vegetable oils they have an extremely high percentage of saturated fatty acids. On the other hand fish oils, which are not a vegetable oil, contain poly and monounsaturated fatty acids.

Fats	*Fatty acid*		
	Saturated	*Mono unsaturated*	*Poly-unsaturated*
Coconut oil	92	6	2
Palm oil	46	44	10
Cotton seed oil	25	25	25
Ground nut oil	19	50	31
Safflower oil	10	15	75
Sunflower oil	8	27	65
Corn oil	8	27	65
Soya bean oil	14	24	62
Butter	60	37	3
Margarine	25	25	50

PSM

Q.4. New drug that prevents a disease but reduce death due to that disease then:

A. Prevalence Increase
B. Prevalence Decrease
C. Incidence Increase
D. Incidence decrease.

Ans: (A)

- Prevalence refers to all current cases (Old and New) existing at a given point in time
- Incidence is the no of new cases occurring in a defined population during a specific period of time.
- **Prevalence = Incidence X duration of time**
- If a new drug not prevent a disease but reduce the death then duration of sickness will increase. But incidence remains the same. So no of diseased persons will increase and prevalence will also increase.

Q.5. Which vaccine should not be kept in freezer:

A. DPT
B. OPV
C. Measles
D. Yellow fever

Ans: (A)

Some Important points about vaccine

- The most heat sensitive vaccine is-***Polio.***
- The vaccines which must be stored in FREEZER compartment are ***1. Polio 2. Measles 3. Yellow fever.***
- Vaccines which must be stored in COLD part but never allowed to freeze are → ***Typhoid, DPT, Tetanus, Toxoid, DT, BCG and DILUENTS.***
- BCG vaccine is reconstituted with ***Normal saline.***
- Measles vaccine is reconstituted with ***distilled water***
- The most popular strain used in measles vaccine is → ***EDMONSTON-ZAGREB.***

- Live vaccines are contraindicated in pregnancy e.g. *Rubella, Yellow fever vaccine.*
- *Meningococcal vaccine*. Recommended after-2 years of Age. No vaccine against- ***Type B strain.***
- In HIV patients for immunization the polio vaccine used is KILLED polio vaccine (*Salk polio vaccine*).
- Measles vaccine once reconstituted with vaccine should be ***used in 1 hour.***
- BCG once reconstituted the vaccine should be used in **3 hour**.

Q.6. Eligible couples are:

A. Husband and wife 15-45 years
B. Wife 15-45 years
C. Newly married couples
D. Men 20-40 years

Ans: (B)

- *Eligible couple*-Refers to currently married couple where, the wife is in the reproductive age between ages of 15 to 45.
- *Target couple*-The couples who have had 2-3 living children and family planning was largely directed to such couples.
- *Couple protection rate*-Defined as the percent of eligible couples effectively protected against childbirth.

(Reference: Park, Page No. 360, 18th Edition)

PSM

Q.7. Fastest population growth in:

A. India
B. Kuwait.
C. Pakistan
D. Sri Lanka

Ans: (A)

Demographic cycle of 5 stages

High stationary

- High birth rate and High death rate which cancel each other.

Early expanding

- High birth rate
- Death rates begin to decline.

Late expanding

- Birth rates begin to fall.
- Death rate declines still further
- **India is in this phase.**

Low Stationary

- Low birth rate
- Low death rate

Declining

- Birth rate % lower than death rate of population begin to decline.

Q.8. Socially acquired behaviour is called as:

A. Custom
B. Socialization
C. Culture
D. Acculturation

Ans: (C)

Culture:

Learned behaviour which has been socially acquired. Culture is the product of human societies.

Customs:

The mere existence of a society, the mere plurality of individuals gives rise to customs from which no single member of the community can escape. Custom are technically divided into **folkways and mores.** The **FOLKWAYS** are right ways of doing things in what is regarded as the less vital areas of human conduct. The more **stringent customs** are called **MORES.**

Socialization:

A process by which an individual gradually acquires culture becomes a member of a social group.

(Reference: Page No. 491, Park, 18th Edition)

Q.9. Upper line in growth chart is:

A. 80th percentile
B. 60th percentile
C. 70th percentile
D. 80th percentile

Ans: (A)

The growth or road to health chart is a visible display of the child's physical growth and development. In India growth chart have 4 reference curves. Topmost curve corresponds to 80% of the median (50th percentile) of the WHO reference standard.

- The lower lines represent to 70%, 60% and 50% of that standard.
- The growth chart recommended by govt. of India shows three degree of MALNUTRITION:
  - 1st degree - **Grade I** or Mild malnutrition-*Child weight: 80-70%*
  - 2nd degree - **Grade II** or Moderate malnutrition-*Child weight: 70-60%*
  - 3rd degree - **Grade III** or Severe malnutrition- *Child weight < 60%*
  - **Grade IV**-*Child weight <50%*

(Reference: Page No. 404, Park, 18th Edition)

Q.10. The family welfare programmer's goal is to reach NRR-1 couple protection rate should be:

A. 20% **B.** 30%
C. 60% **D.** 75%

Ans: (C)

Couple protection rate (CPR) - A couple is considered protected, if one of one of the partners is sterilized or when they are using condom or pills on regular basis or IUD.

- Now the present *CPR - 48 % in India*
- *A CPR of at least 60% is needed to achieve NRR* -1
- Try to remember these point's also.
- IMR per 1000 live birth →56-50
- *Crude birth* rate per 1000 population →23

PSM

- *Crude death* rate per 1000 population ®9
- *Life expectancy*
  Male— 62 years
  Female —63 years

(Reference: Simple Biostatics-Page No. 85, Indrayan.)

Q.11. Which is secondary prevention?

A. Cervix pap smear checking
B. Vaccination
C. Admitting disabled in special schools.
D. Chemoprophylaxis

Ans: (A)

- ***Level of Prevention***
  Primordial Prevention *(prevention of emergency of risk factors).*
- ***Intervention***
  Individual and Mass education. It is a type of primary Intervention.
- **Primary Prevention**
  – *Health Promotion*
  – Health Education
  – Environmental Modification
  – Nutritional Intervention
  – Life style and behaviour changes.
- *Specific Protection*
  – Immunization
  – Chemoprophylaxis
- **Secondary Prevention**
  Early diagnosis and treatment (screening test case finding)
- **Tertiary Prevention**
  Disability limitation and Rehabilitation.

Q.12. Exclusive breastfeeding is recommended by WHO, upto:

A. 3 months
B. 4 months
C. 6 months
D. 9 months

Ans: (C)

PSM

Exclusive breastfeeding:- only breast MILK is given, **no other food or not even water** given. An infant should be exclusively breastfed for 1st 6 months. **Nutritive value of milks compared (Value per 100 gms)**

	Human milk	*Cow milk*
Fat	3.4	4.1
Protein	1.1	3.2
Lactose	7.4	4.4
Ca^{+}	28	120
Iron	—	0.2
Vitamin C	3	1
Minerals	0.1	0.8
Water	88	87
Energy	65	67

Colostrum: The milk secreted during the first 3 days after delivery. The milk contains more antibodies and High amount of vitamin: A, D, E, and K.

(Reference: O.P.Ghai, Page No. 97, 6th Edition/Park, Page No. 445, 18th Edition)

PSM

Q.13. Physical quality of life index includes all *except:*

A. Infant mortality rate (IMR)

B. Expectation of life at one year

C. Literacy rate on population

D. Income

Ans: (D)

PQLI included:
- ➢ IMR
- ➢ Expectation of life at one year.
- ➢ Literacy rate in a population

Human development index included:
- ➢ Education
- ➢ Income
- ➢ Life expectancy.

(Reference: Indryan, Page No. 92)

Q.14. Test which detects the true negative:

A. Specificity

B. Sensitivity
C. Positive predictive value
D. Detect actability

Ans: (A)

Specificity:

- It is the ability of a test to identify correctly who do not have the diseases which is true negative.

Sensitivity:

- It is the ability of a test to identify correctly all those who have the disease which is true positive.

(Reference: Park, Page No. 117,18th Edition)

Q.15. Disease usually not seen in a country but brought from abroad is called:

A. Epizootic.
B. Epornithic
C. Exotic.
D. Endemic

Ans: (C)

1. *Exotic*-Diseases which are imported into a country where they do not otherwise occur, as for example rabies in UK.
2. *Epizootic*-An outbreak (epidemic) of disease in animal population with the implication that it may also affect human population.
3. *Endemic*-It refers to the constant presence of a disease or infection agent with in a given geographical area as population group with out importation from. Outside. May also refer to the usual as expected frequency of the disease with in such area or population group. For instance common cold is endemic because somebody always has one.
4. *Epornithic*-An outbreak of disease in a bird population.
5. *Enzootic*-An epidemic occurring in animal e.g., anthrax, rabies, brucellosis, typhus and tick typhus.

(Reference: Park, Page No. 86,18th Edition)

Q.16. Surveillance is:

A. Continuous Scrutiny.
B. For missing cases.
C. Estimate the incidence rate
D. More costly

Ans: (A)

1. **Surveillance** - is the continue scrutiny of the factors that determine the occurrence and distribution of disease and other condition of all health.
2. **Sentinel Surveillance** - A method for identifying the missing cases and thereby supplementing the modified case is required.

Q.17. Rural community health centre for:

A. 60000 population
B. 30000 population
C. 100000 population
D. 200000 population

Ans: (C)

Please try to remember the following facts:

1. Sub-centre → For 5000 population in general and for 3000 population in hilly and backward areas.
2. PHC caters population of →30000 in general, 20000 hilly, tribal and backward areas.
3. Community health centre → For 80000 to 120000 population.
4. Health assistant (male + female) → For 30000 population in general.
5. Male and female health worker → 5000 in general, and 3000 in hilly areas.
6. Health guide and anganwadi workers → for 1000 population.

(Reference: Park, Page No.696,18th Edition)

Q.18. Best protection from STD and Syphilis:

A. Condom
B. OCP
C. IUCD
D. Diaphragm

Ans: (A)

- Condom provides protection not only against pregnancy but also against STD
- The commonest complication of IUD is *Vaginal Bleeding*
- Male contraceptive pill is - *Gossypol.*
- Femshield (Female condom) - It is known as Fem or femidom. It is newly developed female barrier contraceptive and woman oriented. It is highly protective against spread of STDS and AIDS in particular.

(Reference: Park, Page No. 362, 18th Edition)

Q.19. Multipurpose worker is a:

A. Dai
B. Normal woman
C. Any educated woman
D. Health worker

Ans: (D)

1. One Health worker female and one Health worker male are posted at each sub-centre and cover a population of 5000, they are multipurpose worker.
2. **Dai**-trained for 30 working days.
   The function of Dai:
   – Delivery
   – Health education
   – Registration
   - Health worker: 1 per 5000 population.
   - Trained-dai: One for each village
   - Health assistant: 1 per, 30000 population
   - Anganwadi worker: 1 per 1000 population.

(Reference: Park, Page No. 696, 18th Edition)

Q.20. Temporary contraceptive method of choice in 37-year well educated woman:

A. Diaphragm
B. IUCD
C. Mala-N
D. Mala-D.

Ans: (A)

- <35 year IUCD/pills/other suitable contraceptive methods.
- **> 35 years IUCD is preferred over pills, Specially who are smoker. DMPA or Norplant can be alternative.**
- But this question asked about well educated 37 years old women for temporary contraception. so, Method should be barrier that is **Diaphragm.** Because diaphragm have the advantages of preventing STD, HIV and Reducing the incidence of cancer cervix by preventing viral transmission.

Teen age girl: Low dose pills are most effective for sexually active adolescents. It is contraceptive of choice. However DMPA may be an alternative.

New married couple - Pills are recommended provided there is no contraindication. IUCD should not be preferred because of increase incidence of PID.

Post abortal- pills are ideal.

Post partum-Lactating - Prescribe only after 10 weeks in fully lactating women. Mini pill or inject able steroid if available.

Post partum-Nonlactating - Contraceptive practise should be started after 3 weeks. Pill is good. IUD is an equally effective alternative. Injectable DMPA could be used as it is devoid of any estrogen related side-effects.

- *Barrier method* of contraceptive is best for patients with heart disease.
- IUDs are contraindicated for fear of infection.
- Steroidal contraception is contraindicated in deep vein thrombosis patients.

(Reference:D.C. Dutta Obstetrics-6th Edition, Page Nos. 552, 558)

PSM